Curing Chronic Disease with a Raw, Vegan Diet

Healing With A Raw, Vegan Diet Naturally

by

Dr. Earendil M. Spindelilus D.N.M., M.H., C.R., PSc.D

CURING CHRONIC DISEASE WITH A RAW, VEGAN DIET

COPYRIGHT © 2020 BY EARENDIL M. SPINDELILUS

ALL RIGHTS RESERVED.

PUBLISHED BY TREE OF LIFE HOLISTIC WELLNESS CENTER

COVER ART BY EARENDIL AND PEGGY SPINDELILUS

NO PART OF THIS BOOK MAY BE REPRODUCED IN ANY WRITTEN, ELECTRONIC, RECORDING OR PHOTOGRAPHING WITHOUT WRITTEN PERMISSION OF THE PUBLISHER OR AUTHOR.

FIRST EDITION - **ISBN** - 9798620874606

DISCLAIMER

THIS BOOK IS INTENDED TO PROVIDE INFORMATION ON THE SUBJECT OF CURING CHRONIC DISEASE WITH A RAW, VEGAN DIET. THIS INFORMATION PRESENTED IS NOT INTENDED AS A SUBSTITUTE FOR MEDICAL TRAINING OR ADVICE, BUT EVERY EFFORT HAS BEEN MADE TO ENSURE ACCURACY. THE BOOK IS SOLD WITH THE UNDERSTANDING THAT THE PUBLISHER AND AUTHOR ARE NOT LIABLE FOR ANY MISCONCEPTION OR MISUSE OF THE INFORMATION PROVIDED AND SHALL HAVE NEITHER LIABILITY NOR RESPONSIBILITY TO ANY PERSON OR ENTITY WITH RESPECT TO ANY LOSS, DAMAGE OR INJURY CAUSED OR ALLEGED TO BE CAUSED DIRECTLY OR INDIRECTLY BY THE SAID INFORMATION.

Table of Contents

DEDICATION..5

FORWARD...6

CHAPTER 1 INTRODUCTION...8

CHAPTER 2 WHY RAW, VEGAN?..11

2.1 Why Raw Vegan?..11

2.2 A tale about me..15

2.3 Illnesses directly affected by diet..18

2.4 Nutritional benefits of being raw and vegan..............................24

2.5 How to start..32

2.6 A typical raw kitchen...34

2.7 Beware of adulterated foods..48

CHAPTER 3 RECIPES...53

3.1 Breakfast...53

3.2 Lunch 107

3.3 Entrees..130

3.4 Desserts...194

3.5 Snacks...238

3.6 Salads...261

3.7 Smoothies and juices..285

CHAPTER 4 MENU PLANS...293

4.1 Simple, no equipment needed menus…………………………….…..…293

CHAPTER 5 Actual case histories of healing through a raw, vegan diet…298

5.1 Case History #1………………………………………………………..298

5.2 Case History #2………………………………………………….....301

5.3 Where to go from here …………………………………………….304

ABOUT THE AUTHOR…………………………………………….....311

DEDICATION

To my wife and best friend Peggy, who has stood beside me and put up with all of my time spent getting one degree or certification after another.

To Waya and Sinde, our furry children who love us unconditionally

I would also like to express my gratitude for all of the patients who have taught me so much about how to be a doctor.

Not all doctors are healers and not all healers are doctors.

FORWARD

Would you believe me if I told you that at 48 years old, I have the energy I had in my 20s? Or that my mood is so consistently happy, that almost nothing can touch it? Or that 45 pounds have released from my body in the last 4 months...the 45 pounds that wouldn't budge for nearly 20 years prior no matter what I did? Or that I have nearly eradicated my Lyme Disease and all its painful symptoms after struggling for 20 years? Or that I can't wait to get in my kitchen each day to create the latest raw food delicious masterpiece? Or that I never fell like I'm suffering or missing out on my old "comfort foods" even though I'm eating a raw diet?

I get it because I wouldn't have believed it either! But I'm thrilled to tell you that all of that and more is absolutely true, and it's all because I FINALLY stopped resisting what Dr. S had been nudging me to do for years, and I gave the raw diet a try.

I'm Marci Updyke, and it's my honor and pleasure to introduce you to Dr. S. 20 years ago, I was doing what I loved most, riding my horse at my ranch, when a tick bite resulting in Lyme Disease had staked its claim on my health, vitality, and hope for ever feeling like myself again. In my long search for solutions to relieve the sometimes debilitating symptoms, I experimented with conventional and cutting-edge treatments alike. I did make some progress along the way, but still felt exhausted and frustrated that my life wound have to be on hold every time the awful symptoms returned.

Never giving up my search for solutions, two year ago, I visited the Tree Of Life Holistic Wellness Center and met Dr. S. He recommended the raw diet to me right away, as he felt certain it would help, and he reassured me that it would taste good. "Seriously?" I remember thinking, "How can you make foods in their raw state taste good? What about pizza or Mexican food? Or brownies? I will miss those!" I had already become so restricted with my diet as it was, and I definitely didn't like the idea of restricting myself even more. Plus I guess I didn't feel "sick enough" to go to such extremes, so I graciously declined, "Thanks but no thanks, Dr. S."

Another eighteen months passed and my Lyme symptoms became activated again. I was so sick that time, that I was willing to do anything to feel better. That's when I remember Dr. S tell me about the raw diet. I decided, "It's time. I've tried everything else. What do I have to lose?"

So I started researching raw recipes and trying to recreate all my favorite foods. And guess what? Dr. S was right! Eating raw DOES taste good. But even more exciting than that, I started noticing my unleashed energy that was different from a temporary coffee buzz and thought, "Oh my gosh! Where in the heck did all this energy come from?" I found myself bouncing out of bed without an alarm with energy that doesn't quit all day. After only 4 months, I truly have gotten what I never thought was possible – my LIFE BACK.

I am so beyond grateful for Dr. S for guiding me here. The only regret I have is that I didn't listen to him sooner, because this was the best decision I've ever made.

So what does this mean for you? Well, maybe you don't have Lyme Disease, but maybe you're not feeling that great. Maybe you're starting to believe that getting older means that it's normal to lose energy, gain weight, and feel like you're dragging yourself around all day just waiting for the day to be over. Well, I'm here to tell you that it doesn't have to be like that! If I can feel this incredible with Lyme Disease, then SURELY you can feel amazing too!

I believe we all need a nudge sometimes, like Dr. S gave me. So here's my nudge to you. Just try a raw diet for 30 days and see for yourself. Think about it: What do you have to lose? Nothing! But you have health and vitality to gain.

CHAPTER 1

Introduction

"Let your food be your medicine and your medicine be your food"
Hippocrates

A vegan diet is now considered the fastest growing lifestyle change in the United States. There are now estimated to be approximately 1.6 million currently who call themselves vegan in America, up 600%.

According to Food Revolution Network: First of all, according to a forecast report by restaurant consultancy group Baum + Whiteman in New York, *"plant-based" will be the food trend of 2018*. The report also anticipates that **plant-based foods will become the new organic**.

In addition, Nestlé, **the largest food company in the world,** predicts **that plant-based foods will continue to grow and … this trend is "here to stay."**

Another company, international delivery service Just Eat named *veganism as a top consumer trend in 2018* — due to a 94% increase in "healthy food ordered."

And similarly, according to data released by GrubHub, the top takeaway marketplace in the U.S., orders for plant-based food have reached a new high. In particular, users *chose vegan food 19% more* in the first half of 2017 than in the first half of 2016.

In the UK, the number of people identifying as vegans has increased by 350%, compared to a decade ago, according to research commissioned by the Vegan Society in partnership with Vegan Life magazine.

In Portugal, **vegetarianism rose by 400% in the last decade**. This is according to research carried out by Nielsen.

In Australia, between 2014 and 2016, the number of food products launched carrying a vegan claim **rose by 92%**. And **Australia is the third-fastest growing vegan market in the world.**

Mainstream health organizations are recommending a plant-based diet. Including, among others: Kaiser Permanente, the largest healthcare organization in the U.S.; the Dietary Guidelines Advisory Committee; and the American Institute for Cancer Research.

Even Walmart, the world's largest retailer, is asking **its suppliers to offer more plant-based products!**

So, an understandable question would be … why? Why such a fast growth pattern in a world still rife with animal factory farming and meat based traditions?

For some, the choice is a compassionate one. They simply do not want to eat other animals when their dietary requirements do not need them to die.

But, for most, the choice is one based on health concerns. According to www.pwc.com Chronic diseases and conditions are on the rise worldwide. An aging population and changes in societal behavior are contributing to a steady increase in these common and costly long-term health problems.

The middle class is growing; and with urbanisation accelerating, people are adopting a more sedentary lifestyle. This is pushing obesity rates and cases of diseases such as diabetes upward. According to the World Health Organization, chronic disease prevalence is expected to rise by 57% by the year 2020. Emerging markets will be hardest hit, as population growth is anticipated be most significant in developing nations. Increased demand on healthcare systems due to chronic disease has become a major concern.

For many people, there was a time when switching to a vegan diet was very difficult, in part due to the lack of nutritional education in this country, but also due to a lack of food options and recipes out there. Fortunately, this has changed much for the better.

For example, when I first went vegan, there were few food options as vegan substitutes. Not any more. When the website veganessentials.com first was created they probably had about 20 food products, mostly a few fake meats. Now they boast approximately 1500 products, ranging from main meals, snacks, desserts, etc.

For recipes the go to site is vegweb.com. Again, when they first came out they had a couple of hundred recipes or so, Now, you can find 15,000 online under about any category you can imagine.

The science has also come a long way, with more and more third party, independent trial studies being done proving the efficacy of a plant-based diet. Finally, more and more doctors are coming on board promoting this new lifestyle change with such famous names as Dr. Kim A. Williams M.D., Dr. T. Colin Cambell phD., Dr. Caldwell Esselstyn, M.D., Angie Sadeghi, M.D., Dr. John A. McDougall, M.D., Dr. Dean Ornish, M.D., Dr. Neal Barnard, M.D., Dr. Brooke Goldner, M.D., Dr. Michael Greger, M.D., Dr. Michael Klaper, M.D., Dr. Joel Kahn, M.D., Dr. Pamela A. Popper, phD., Garth Davis, M.D., Dr. Alan Goldhamer, D.C., Dr. Ellsworth Wareham, M.D. and so MANY more.

So, lets see what all the hullabaloo is about and what it takes to accomplish this in our own lives, by starting with a small explanation of why raw and my story ...

CHAPTER 2

Why Raw, Vegan?

2.1 Why raw, vegan?

I would like to start off stating it is my belief that, the body given the opportunity, can heal from anything. This said, each person's situation is unique and may require more or less of an effort on their part. I seen some wonderful healing occur but it is up to the individual to be a significant part of the process.

One of the most, if not the most, important change that I would do is the change to a vegan diet during the healing process, especially one with little processed foods, thereby utilizing significantly raw fruits and vegetables and sprouted nuts and grains. This allows the body to heal without having to deal with the energy of digesting heavily processed foods and thereby directing the body's resources to healing the matters at hand. It also floods the body with a vast amount of micro-nutrients, thereby giving the system what it needs to rebuild. The first step to any healing is Cleanse and Nourish. Raw food enthusiasts claim that a raw diet increases energy levels, facilitates weight loss and improves overall health.

A raw food diet incorporates only uncooked foods that undergo no processing. The raw meal plan allows dieters to avoid high concentrations of unhealthy fats and excessive sugar often found in processed supermarket foods. Features The key principle guiding a raw food diet is to consume foods only in their most natural states. According to website RawFoodLife.com, a food can only be considered uncooked if it has never been heated above 118 degrees Fahrenheit.

A raw food diet also requires that fruits and vegetables be raw, unaltered and additive-free. This guideline means that raw food dieters must eat only organic produce that is not genetically modified or treated with pesticides.

Raw food dieters cannot drink alcohol or modified beverages, included pasteurized milk. Instead, drink raw cashew milk or raw almond milk if it is available. Consider making your own juices out of raw oranges, apples or vegetables. Nutrition Raw foods are naturally full of important dietary vitamins and minerals. The website WeLikeItRaw.com emphasizes the importance of leafy green vegetables such as lettuce, spinach, broccoli, kale or mustard greens. These are sources of folate, iron, calcium and vitamins A, C and K. Include sugary fruits as well as unprocessed foods high in unsaturated fats. Avocados, nuts, seeds and olives are energy-rich foods that adhere to raw food guidelines.

Benefits: People who adhere to a raw food diet claim that it boosts their energy levels, improves immune functioning, helps them lose weight and cleanses their bodies. According to RawFoodLife.com, a raw diet increases the body's pH levels, making it more alkaline and increasing its energy. Raw diet proponents also claim that cooking destroys a food's natural enzymes -- components important for nutrition. A diet high in fruits and vegetables does contain many important vitamins and minerals lacking in a number of processed foods. Raw Food Meals For an example of a balanced week-long raw food diet, WeLikeItRaw.com recommends eating sugar-rich fruits such as melons, oranges or apples for breakfast. A smoothie incorporating bananas and other fruits is an excellent way to incorporate healthy, raw fruits into your diet.

For lunch and dinner, eat a large salad composed of a variety of leafy greens. Include avocados, nuts, seeds and other fat-rich raw foods to boost your energy levels. Avoid processed salad dressings in favor of a blended dressing composed of an avocado and an orange or lemon.
For snacks, eat one or two servings of fruit. These provide carbohydrates that improve your energy level throughout the day. Supplement meals with dried fruits, nuts or raw vegetables.

How to Eat:
• Eat only when hungry and never overeat.
• Turn off the television and radio.
• Sit down to eat.
• Eat slowly and deliberately chewing each mouthful thoroughly.
• Don't talk and don't be bothered by any distractions.

- Thank your higher power for every bite, and give thanks before and after each meal.

You'd be surprised who's listening and the powers they/he/she/it can infuse into your food. We are spiritual beings experiencing a physical reality. Bring the spirit to your table.

Shopping suggestions: Knowing what foods and how much you will need from the grocery store for the week can be confusing when you are starting a raw food diet plan, so it is helpful to have a well planned out shopping list. If you don't think ahead, you very well may end up hitting the super market every day or worse, succumbing to eating cooked foods if the refrigerator is lacking raw foods. Use your meal plans to estimate how much fruit you will need. Buying a lot of raw food can also take a hit on your wallet if you do not learn how to be thrifty in the produce aisles, so remember these tips and you will become an expert raw food shopper. 1. Shop for 5 days worth I have found that if I try to shop for a full weeks worth of food that I will have rotting food, an overstuffed refrigerator, and will end up running back to the store only for certain items. 2. Load up on bananas and watermelon.

Buy a lot of these fruits because they are cheap, keep well, and are high in calories. I like to buy some bananas ripe and some green so that by the time I am done eating the ripe ones, the green ones are ready for me. If you notice some overly ripe bananas are on the verge of rotting then peel them and freeze them for future smoothies or "ice cream". 3. Buy berries on sale Berries, especially organic, tend to be very expensive and low in calories for a raw food diet plan that relies on high calorie sweet fruits, so I rarely bother with them. If I want some for smoothies, I usually buy them frozen or wait for a sale. 4. On buying greens For 5 days worth of raw food diet plan meals,

I purchase 5 pounds of greens, being careful to choose different varieties so that my body gets the full spectrum of what nature has to offer. Baby greens, arugula, romaine, and iceberg are all good picks. Although I am not proud of my plastic usage, the pre-packaged greens tend to be less expensive than the loose greens. 5. Look for deals In the summer it is MUCH cheaper to shop at produce stands than a grocery store and year round produce is usually less expensive at health food stores, although their selection is often more meager. Sometimes you can even seek to arrange a deal where you can receive older produce for a lesser fee or even for free, when these foods would otherwise be thrown out. 6. Stock up on dried fruit Having dried fruit on hand is great for a late evening snack or something quick to grab when running out the door. Best of all, it keeps for a long time so if you run out of fruit you will have something to hold you over. Sun dried fruits are best and be careful there are no preservatives added. Sprouts and sprouted grains show up frequently in raw food diets.

Raw food cookbook author Ani Phyo points out that, although raw foodies do not tend to consume highly processed foods, they can create remarkably creative recipes from raw ingredients such as sprouts. Her recipe of sprouted rice with wild corn and tomato spikes the concoction with cilantro, garlic and jalapeno pepper. Many raw foodies sprout their own lentils and grains and use them in salads and raw bread recipes.

2.2 A tale about me

As a very young child I believe my family found me quite odd. While most children my age were out playing baseball, hide and go seek and such, I was out roaming the forests near our home looking for the secrets hidden therein. One of my passions was how to heal using the natural world. At 12 years of age I founded a club where I could teach my young friends how to identify and find various herbs and other plants growing in our area. We would talk about their healing properties and would learn to make various teas and such from them. A bit nerdy perhaps?

With these early lessons I became aware of how important our health was and how nature could play such a significant role in it. As a child I had a tendency to get colds quite a bit and I was that child who went to school with a raw upper lip from blowing my nose so frequently. This would happen multiple times a year, year in and year out.

I eventually began my formal schooling in holistic medicine and a significant part of it included nutrition. I had always felt it was wrong to eat animal products, from a compassionate point of view so it was easy to accept the nutritional benefits of going more plant-based. So, at 22 years old, mainly due to compassion for other animals, I became a vegetarian. At that time we did not know of the word vegan. I was no longer eating any form of animal flesh though I still had dairy and products that contained eggs.

At that point I noticed a significant change in my health. While I still became sick at least a couple of times a year, the colds were less severe and I had so much more energy.

Ten years passed and I learned more about nutrition and my compassion side kicked in more, so by the age of 32 I became a full-fledged, card carrying vegan. My wife and I were sitting in a Pizza Hut on the beach in Gulf Shores Alabama and I was eating a cheese pizza. Something clicked within me and I looked at my wife and told her this was my last one. I figured at that time I would never taste anything like a cheese pizza again. Back then the selection and availability of vegan foods was pretty sparse and most of what you ate needed to be home cooked. There were few vegan restaurants and certainly no vegan pizzas.

Again, I noticed a quantum leap in my health, a nice side-effect to compassion. Now I only became sick about once a year. I had part of my formal education completed and I was finally running my own practice. A common statistic with doctors in private practice, especially those in a clinical environment is that they become sick quite frequently, in part due to stress as well as to exposure with the patients. To combat this I would take three to five cloves of garlic, pressed and swallow them each morning, seven days a week, 365 days a year. It is a well known medical fact that three to five cloves of garlic has the same efficacy as an adult dose of penicillin, without destroying your micro-flora balance. This helped quite a bit warding off the multitude of colds and flu that entered the clinic each day. But I would still occasionally get sick.

Finally, after about 15 years of being vegan I decided to try my hand at a raw, vegan diet. I had already studied extensively and I knew of the benefits of having a diet rich in active enzymes and micro-nutrients. One of my main problems with this was simply that my wife is an amazing vegan cook. You name it and she is able to make a wonderful vegan version of it. Even at parties full of meat eaters hers was the dish first devoured.

But, there came a time when I simply did not like the "dense" feelings I had. As you change your diet and you cleanse naturally on healthy foods, you become more sensitive and aware of your body and how it feels on certain foods. I began to notice that I did not have that light, healthy energy I felt I should be having each day. So, in spite of my wife's excellent cooking skills, I took the plunge and went 100% raw. Even I was surprised at the changes that occurred so quickly.

In a couple of weeks my weight dropped down to a more comfortable range. For years I had experienced a severe issue with mold sensitivity and after a month that problem had resolved itself. Even my allergy to poison oak disappeared. I no longer needed to take the garlic each morning as I was not affected by the patient's issues. Since then, I have not experienced any illness. My sleep issues have also completely disappeared and I find sleep the gentle, healing process it was meant to be. As a side benefit to my wife, my snoring issue was also completely alleviated and her nights are gentler as well.

I have since then stayed on the raw, vegan diet and my health has yet to plateau. Each day I feel more energy and endurance than I can remember ever experiencing before. I have found I need to eat only one meal a day with a few raw snacks in the evening. I rarely get hungry and I have plenty of energy before I ever have my main meal of the day.

I now tell my patients about this diet routine and some of them are trying to switch, especially my cancer patients. As they progress in the program utilizing more and more of a raw, vegan diet we have found that their healing process is greatly accelerated and the medications we have them on are more effective. We are also teaching classes on nutrition with an emphasis on a raw, vegan diet.

Myself on Mt Shasta 8000 Feet snowshoeing before our first meal of the day.

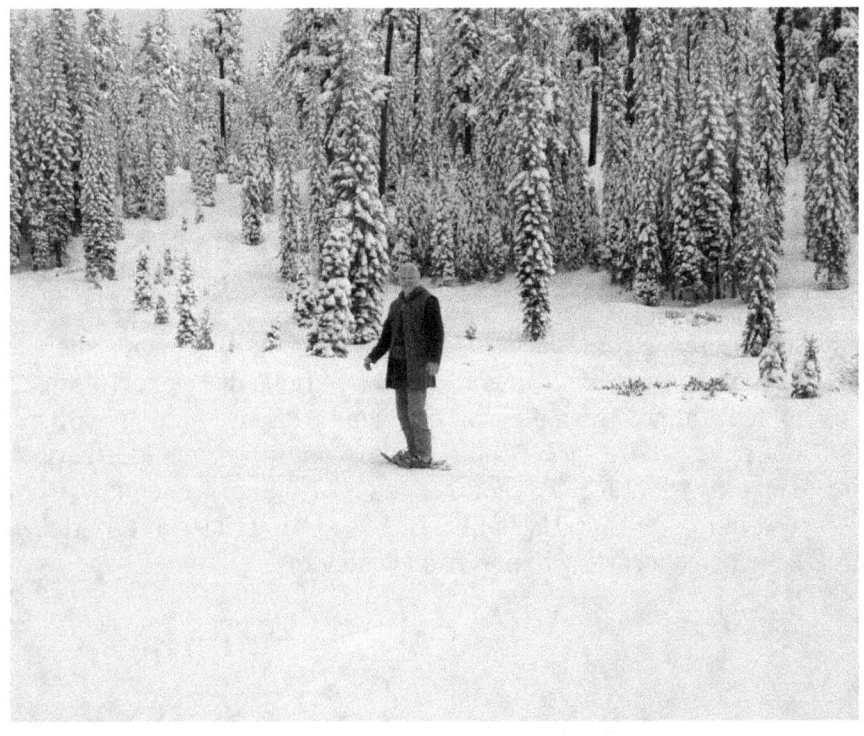

2.3 Illnesses directly affected by diet

According to the website usrtk.org: Americans suffer from an epidemic of food-related diseases, such as obesity; type 2 diabetes; cardiovascular, liver and kidney diseases; some types of cancer, and Alzheimer's disease.

The U.S. government estimates that about half of all American adults—117 million people—have one or more preventable, chronic diseases, many of which are related to poor quality eating patterns and physical inactivity. Rates of these chronic, diet-related diseases continue to rise.

These diseases are caused, in part, by a food industry that promotes processed food packed with unhealthy ingredients, including high fructose corn syrup, added sugars, trans fats, artificial sweeteners, artificial flavors and colors, preservatives and other additives.

According to The Cancer Project, at least a third of yearly cancer deaths in the U.S. can be attributed to dietary factors. Their review of various scientific studies estimated that up to 80 percent of cancers of the large bowel, breast, and prostate result from dietary factors. It's also suspected that due to an increase in our consumption of animal products, we're also consuming a greater number of carcinogens found in animal tissues and milk.

Dietary guidance issued by U.S. Department of Health and Human Services and the U.S. Department of Agriculture are often politicized and polarized, with industry influence trumping science and the government's own health advisers.

According to reference.com: lack of sufficient dietary elements such as proteins, vitamins and nutrient minerals causes various deficiency diseases, according to Healthline. Examples of deficiency diseases along with the respective nutrients whose lack results in the conditions include: beriberi (vitamin B1), kwashiorkor (protein), goiter (iodine), anemia (iron), marasmus (protein), pellagra (vitamin B3), scurvy (vitamin C), rickets (vitamin D) and osteoporosis (vitamin D and calcium).

Deficiency diseases

- Diseases caused due to deficiency of nutrients of our food.
- Examples:
i. Proteins deficiency diseases
ii. Carbohydrates deficiency diseases
iii. Vitamins deficiency diseases
iv. Minerals deficiency diseases

Nutrient deficiencies lead to an array of diseases and health conditions, including dementia and death, explains Healthline. Vitamin deficiencies are associated with several deficiency diseases, underscoring the need to ensure sufficient vitamin intake. Mineral deficiencies are also associated with diseases, including goiter, rickets and anemia. A nutritional deficiency can be caused by intake of inadequate nutrients, or a defect in the body's absorption mechanism.

With the increasing rate of chronic diseases there have been more and more studies done as to finding the root cause of this trend. Time after time nutrition is found to be a significant contributing factor. According to the U.S. Department of Agriculture, the type and quantity of food or beverages you consume can have a significant effect on your health. In some cases, the food you eat may cause certain diseases or symptoms to manifest. Diet-related diseases can affect most of your body's systems, depending on your specific disease. Diet-related diseases can be mild, moderate or severe.

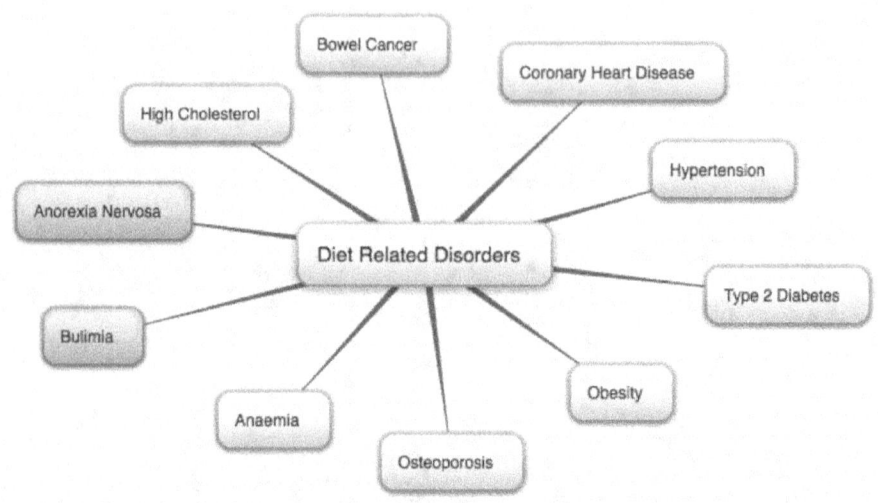

A short list of some of these diseases:

- Celiac
- Acne Vulgaris
- Irritable Bowel Syndrome
- Lucrative Colitis
- Cancer
- Hypertension
- Cholesterol
- Osteoporosis
- Allergies
- Heart Disease
- Candida (Leaky gut)
- Anemia
- Headaches and migraines
- Obesity
- Diabetes (both type 1 and 2)
- Stroke
- Gout
- Gallbladder diseases and gallstones.
- Kidney stones
- Arthritis

- Pulmonary disorders
- Asthma
- Acid reflux
- COPD

Needless to say, I can go on, and on ...

A great website I love to go to is www.pcrm.org which is the Physicians Committee for Responsible Medicine. As they put it so well "People following vegan diets are less likely to develop chronic diseases, compared with other dietary groups, according to a study funded by the NIH/National Cancer Institute. Researchers analyzed the diets of those following vegan, lacto-ovo-vegetarian, semi-vegetarian, pesco-vegetarian, and non-vegetarian eating patterns and tracked several health biomarkers. Based on those biomarkers, the vegan group had the lowest risk for cancer, heart disease, and hypertension, compared with the other groups.

The vegan group also had higher levels of omega-3 fatty acids and higher serum levels of carotenoids and isoflavones associated with lower inflammation. Vegans consumed the most fruits, vegetables, whole grains, and legumes and had the highest intakes of beta-carotene and fiber and the lowest intakes of saturated fatty acids. The vegan group was the only group to be in a healthy weight range, while all other groups were overweight, on average. These findings offer more insight into the relationship between diet-related biomarkers and disease and support vegan diets as a healthful approach to disease prevention."

A randomized controlled study conducted by PCRM, George Washington University and the University of Toronto discovered that subjects placed on a vegan diet had "significantly greater reductions" in their hemoglobin A1c, weight, LDL ("harmful" cholesterol) and body mass index compared to subjects who followed dietary guidelines issued by the American Diabetes Association. "I hope this study will rekindle interest in using diet changes first, rather than prescription drugs," Barnard said.

Vegan diets appear to help with shedding unwanted pounds and maintaining a healthy weight. A 2009 study completed by physician Laurie Barclay suggested that plant-based diets protect against obesity. Two years earlier, the September 2007 journal Obesity, published a study entitled "A Two-Year Randomized Weight Loss Trial Comparing a Vegan Diet to a More Moderate Low-Fat Diet." The study determined that subjects placed on the vegan diet showed significantly greater weight loss than individuals on a standard low-fat weight reduction plan.

Kaiser (leading health insurance company) recommends Vegan diet

- Physicians should consider recommending a plant-based diet to all their patients, especially those with high blood pressure, diabetes, cardiovascular disease, or obesity
- This may also **reduce the number of medications** needed to treat chronic diseases and lower ischemic heart disease mortality rates

EPIC-Oxford study

- Non-meat eaters, **especially vegans**, have a lower prevalence of hypertension and lower systolic and diastolic blood pressures than meat eaters

In his book, *Get Healthy, Go Vegan,** physician Neal Barnard made an astonishing observation regarding how diet impacts our health. According to Barnard, meals laden with meat and dairy have caused a surge in cancer, heart disease, diabetes, obesity and other life-threatening ailments.

But Barnard and several other highly respected physicians, scientists and dieticians are pointing to studies that say we have the ability to reverse and even prevent many illnesses by eliminating all animal products. Organizations like the **Physician's Committee for Responsible Medicine** (PCRM) have even collected scientific data proving that meat and dairy are major contributors to disease, while wholesome fresh fruits, vegetables, grains and soy products may play a major role in warding off various diseases such as cancer.

Consuming soy products like tofu may also boost the efficacy of traditional cancer therapies. A 1999 study by M.F. McCarty appearing in Nutrition revealed that "soy protein, as well as many other vegan proteins, are higher in non-essential amino acids than most animal-derived food proteins," and could possibly offer greater health benefits.

Famed Harvard-trained physician and researcher Dean Ornish studied a group of heart patients who were place on low-fat, plant-based diets. Ornish reported that day-by-day the patients' coronary arteries gradually widened and caused chest pain to "dissolve almost like magic."

2.4 Nutritional benefits of being raw and vegan

For myself, I have seen how my health has changed over the years and I have yet to plateau, in other words to find my peak health, as each day I continue to feel more energy and health than ever before in my life. A wonderful explanation of the some of the health benefits of a raw, vegan are listed with **www.evolvingwellness.com**:

1. Makes You More Health Conscious

It is almost impossible to be a raw vegan and not be health-conscious. In fact, a raw vegan dietary approach tends to make people the most aware, conscious, and mindful about their food choices, compared to any other dietary approach. Those who follow this approach are not only intentional about what food they are eating but typically about the source of that food and its quality as well.

People who are raw vegan aren't only more conscientious about their food but tend to adopt overall, healthier lifestyle habits, and be more mindful of all of their lifestyle choices, and how any of these choices impact the health of our Earth.

2. Helps You Avoid Processed Food

Unlike regular veganism, raw veganism adheres and refers most specifically to *whole food* and *clean eating*. A person who is just vegan can easily eat lots of processed and unhealthy foods, but if you are raw vegan, then nearly all, if not all, of the foods you eat, will typically be whole, real, unrefined, and unprocessed. All processed foods involve some thermal treatment during their processing, like high-heat cooking, roasting, pasteurization, etc. All of this processing strips the food of so much of its beneficial attributes while introducing many harmful properties. (This all applies to home-cooking of foods at high temperatures or for prolonged periods of time as well.)

And unfortunately most processed foods today are made up of ingredients that are themselves refined, processed, or synthetic, leading to a final product that is far removed from being any kind of nourishing or healthful substance. Therefore, a raw vegan approach helps a person automatically (and easily) avoid the thousands of unnatural additives that are found in our "food" today, effectively decreasing the stress and toxic load on the body. These include refined sugars and oils, genetically modified organisms, colors and flavors, synthetic vitamins and minerals, preservatives and other food additives, which are all linked to health problems in numerous ways.

3. Offers the Highest Nutrient Density

When veganism is done via whole, real plant foods, it offers us the highest nutrient density and the lowest amount of problems, as related to our food. There is ample research showing how overall plant-based diets are the most healing and protective. This can be further increased by raw veganism, given the overall negative attributes of heavily heat-treated food.

Most plant foods are the highest in nutrients and the lowest in calories. These foods are also the richest in heat-sensitive nutrients, though really all nutrients are impacted by heat in one way or another. This includes carbohydrates, proteins, fats, vitamins, minerals, antioxidants, and phytonutrients. (Low heat for short time = least destructive; high heat for a long time = most destructive.)

4. Offers a Diet Naturally High in Fruits and Vegetables

The diets of raw vegans have a high composition of fruits and vegetables, which are the most healing, preventative, protective, and valuable foods on Earth. All plant foods provide lots of wholesome vitamins and minerals, as well as phytonutrients and some antioxidants, but fruits and vegetables specifically excel in all of these areas. In addition, they are loaded with fiber and naturally ultra-low in sodium and fat.

Diets high in fruits and vegetables are most beneficial for healing and protecting us from pretty much every diseased condition, including cancers, heart disease, diabetes, arthritis, osteoporosis, infections, as well as cognitive and age-related degenerative diseases. They also support optimal mental and emotional health and well-being.

5. Offers a Diet Naturally High in Fiber

Being solely based on plant foods, the diets of raw vegans are exceptionally high in fiber, which has numerous health and healing attributes. Fiber provides bulk; this helps to optimize satiety and intestinal health. It keeps our intestines clean by collecting, moving, and removing waste along in a timely manner. This, in turn, keeps our elimination regular, which is one of the most important detoxification mechanisms of our body. (Those who eat natural, high-fiber diets typically have healthy bowel movements more than once each day.)

Fiber also acts as a prebiotic, optimizing the healthy and beneficial microflora (microbes) of our intestines. While most people are preoccupied with probiotics, not enough understand the value and importance of prebiotics. We can keep putting in supplemental probiotics religiously, but if our intestines do not provide a hospitable environment for them, they are of little use and benefit to us. This is where prebiotics, via fiber-rich, whole plant foods excel again.

The benefits of diets high in fiber include optimal blood sugar, cholesterol, and blood pressure regulation, decreased risk of colon cancer and protection from cancer, decreased risk of heart disease, and increased longevity. Fiber also helps us lose weight effectively, and sustainably maintain a healthy weight for our body.

6. Offers the Most Alkalizing Diet

The acid-alkaline balance is one of the most vital components for health and wellbeing, yet it is still one of the least emphasized and appreciated health topics. In a nutshell, our body's overall biochemistry is slightly alkaline (basic), with reference to the blood. Your blood must stay in a tightly controlled pH range of roughly 7.4 for you to be healthy, and stay alive. Everything that enters the blood influences the blood pH, though our body will do everything in its power to keep that blood pH slightly alkaline.

So what are the most alkalizing foods? Fruits and vegetables. Diets high in fruits and vegetables, as is the foundation for raw vegan diets, are therefore the most alkalizing. Not only do they contain the most of the "right foods" but they also contain the least or none of the "wrong foods" — the most acidic foods: animal protein and refined carbohydrates. As I share in my book **Healing & Prevention Through Nutrition**, a proper acid-alkaline balance is associated with a decreased risk of and strongest protection against lifestyle diseases like cancer, heart disease, and osteoporosis. It is essential for optimal immune function, decreasing or altogether eliminating our susceptibility to infections, and optimal weight maintenance.

7. Offers Most Support for Beneficial Enzymes

Living bodies and living foods contain enzymes; cells require enzymes to survive and function. Enzymes are biological catalysts, which help to bring about and increase the speed of essential reactions. Even though enzymes are known to withstand the reactions they catalyze, they can become damaged, destroyed, and depleted. Over time, poor diets, which are high in processed and animal food, stress, smoking, and similar negative lifestyle factors catch up to us, and one of the most common results is poor digestion and systemic inflammation. The result is sometimes referred to as enzyme exhaustion, which results in poor health, increased aging and/or decreased longevity.

So how can the raw vegan diet benefit us in this regard? Like most other biological compounds, enzymes are sensitive to various conditions, including temperature and pH. To maintain the integrity of enzymes, temperatures should be kept below 48C/118F. Of course, typical cooking is done at temperatures higher than this. (For reference, the temperature of boiling water is 100C/212F, and baking is done above temperatures of 150C/300F.) This means the destruction of not only the enzymes found in our living plant foods, but as mentioned earlier, a denaturation of most (if not all) nutrients to some degree. In his book Enzyme Nutrition, leading enzyme researcher, the late Dr. Edward Howell also explains the mechanism by which raw foods decrease the exhaustive load on our body's enzymes, by essentially coming in with their own "tools" to help the digestion process.

8. Offers Most Support for Life Energy

Amongst all diets, the diets of raw vegans provide the highest amount of life energy. [Please note that life energy from food is not the same as caloric energy.] All living beings contain life energy — you, me, other animals, plants, etc. This is our essence, the foundation of life, and is known as "Chi", "Qi", "life force", or "prana". Life energy is literally the key to life and not something that needs to be proved but simply experienced. Holistically-oriented disciplines like *Traditional Chinese Medicine* understand its importance, our reductionist science, unfortunately, does not. We are born with abundant life energy and as we go through life that energy fluctuates, increasing or decreasing, depending on our lifestyle choices. When life energy becomes too depleted or blocked, from a metaphysical stance, this is what creates fatigue, ill-feeling or disease.

Everything in our life has an impact on our life energy—it will either enhance, deplete, or provide a neutral effect on it. The same goes for food, which is one of the biggest reasons why those who are spiritually-attuned often turn towards a raw vegan diet, as raw vegan food is "living food" and has the highest potential of life energy. When an animal is killed, its life energy is destroyed, and so eating meat for example by its very nature is eating "dead food". On the other hand, when plants are picked for food, they are still alive and contain life energy. As they age (in the store or on the counter), or are processed, or cooked, their life energy begins to diminish or becomes destroyed, to the point that any plant food that has been heavily cooked or processed is also considered "dead" food. Kirlian photography can exemplify some of this visually, as it can show the bio-energetic field of the food.

The practical consequences of this are that most raw vegans benefit from excellent energy, mental clarity, and vitality levels, as compared to the majority of the public, who are lethargic and plagued with fatigue, mental fog, and disease. Raw vegan diets are simply put highly energizing—high-frequency diets. However, life energy also influences our emotional, mental, and spiritual health, as well as longevity, creativity, and overall wellbeing. This is just another reason why it is common to experience profound surges in these areas as a raw vegan.

9. Increases Consumption of the Optimal Form of Foods

As we establish a fresh relationship with our food, a natural consequence and benefit of the raw vegan path is to consume food in its most optimal form. For fruits and vegetables, this is easy, as they can easily be consumed just as they are. For nuts, seeds, grains, and beans, it is a little different.

Nuts, seeds, grains, and beans are all botanical seeds. As such, they have two main phases to their life-cycle: a dry, dormant one and a wet, living one. The differentiating factor is the presence or absence of water. As we all know, water is essential for life, and it serves as the main catalyst to bring dry, dormant seeds into the living phase. As such, the biochemical makeup of the seed changes. Upon soaking and/or sprouting the seed's nutrient inhibitors are neutralized/diminished, while its various life-giving processes and nutrients are activated and increased. This process begins the growth of new life, activating enzymes, higher nutrient-density, and life energy. As you can imagine, this translates to even more benefits of these foods for us, than if they are just eaten in their dry or cooked forms.

10. Avoids Problems Associated with Animal Foods

All vegans, raw or not, avoid problems related to animal foods, including meat/seafood, dairy, and eggs, regardless of how they are farmed or sourced. The problems associated with these foods go above and beyond our health and the environment. Although it is great that more emphasis is placed today on how destructive animal foods are to our personal health and that of the Earth, many people are completely unaware of the more subtle, yet all-encompassing, problems related to these foods. These include mental, emotional, social, and spiritual.

11. Supports Optimal Digestion for Optimal Longevity

Digestion is a taxing process and the more we eat, and the worse we eat, the more digestive problems and other health problems we tend to encounter. For example: the harder the foods are to digest (i.e. meat), or the more undesirable qualities they bring with them (i.e. processed food), the more we literally "wear" out our body. However as I mentioned in earlier parts of this article, cooked foods add in their own slew of problems that can interfere with optimal health, and thus longevity.

Raw vegan diets provide the body the food in its most natural form. And although some experts or laypeople alike argue that cooked food is easier to digest, which in some ways it is, I feel it is rather naive for us to think that our body wasn't designed to best handle food in its raw and natural form. The fact that we have conditioned ourselves into cooked foods, and today many people whose diets are based on cooked foods have a hard time digesting raw foods is a whole other story. Unhealthy gut flora, backed up intestines, sluggish or stressed out organs, chronic acidity, chronic dehydration, chronic infections, and the like, are just a few of the areas that can interfere with optimal digestion.

Additionally, the diets of raw vegans tend to be naturally lower in calories, since raw vegan food is predominantly rich in nutrients, not calories. This connects us back to the outstanding health benefits of nutrient density we talked about above. People, therefore, tend to eat less, as the body is getting all that it needs more efficiently, and this translates to greater longevity benefits.

12. Financial Benefits

In addition to all of the above health and nutrition benefits, a raw vegan approach also offers some outstanding economical benefits. At first glance, people often rate the raw vegan diet as more expensive. But the question we need to ask ourselves is, compared to what? If comparing it to a diet based on highly processed food, especially refined carbohydrates and fast foods (think Kraft dinner, burgers, fries, soda, and chips), then yes it will be more expensive, but that really isn't a fair comparison as the other stuff isn't even real food. On the other hand, we compare raw veganism to a whole-food omnivore diet, then it can easily come out cheaper. An average meal can easily be $3 (or less) per adult, as I have discovered daily in my life over the past several years.

What else we need to take into consideration here is that both cooked vegan and omnivore diets require just that: cooking. Consider the number of hours each household may spend on running the stove-top, oven, toaster, toaster oven, grill or barbecue, and similar appliances, and how this stacks up the financial costs of such diets. We can also add in the variety of cookware required and how much the mentioned appliances add up to costing us on their own. Factor in the lower environmental and health costs associated with raw vegan diets and the benefits just keep stacking up.

The economic benefits, however, are just one part of this equation. From a practical perspective, raw vegan meal preparation can also be one of the easiest, quickest, and simplest. Of course, this will all depend on us—our personal approach, motivation, ambition, education, creativity, and habits, as to whether we get the most or the least benefits from the raw vegan diet.

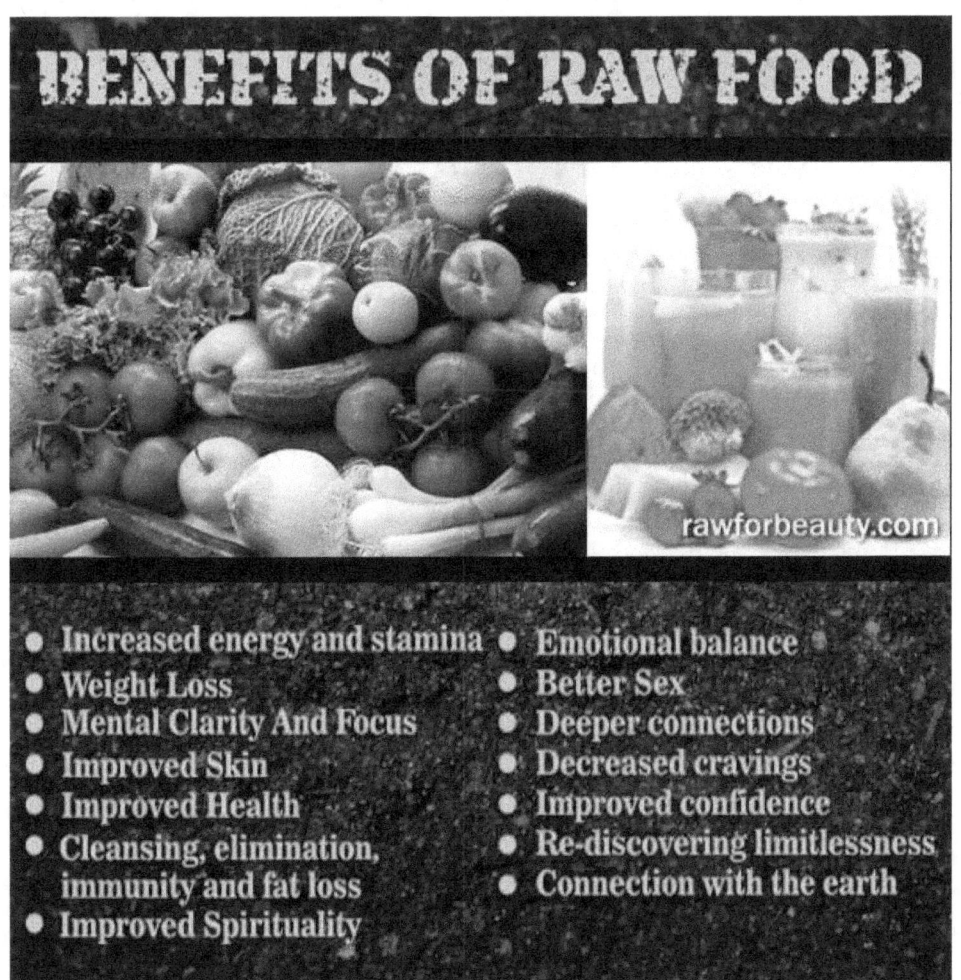

2.5 How to start

When getting started with a new raw vegan diet, what could be more important than simply having plenty of food around? Since you are going to be making a whole lot of food at home now, you'll need to make a special trip to the market to stock your pantry with all the fun new ingredients of your diet! Peruse your new raw recipe books for all those exciting new words like nama shoyu, wakame, and agave nectar. Over time you can build up your collection of spices, nuts, and seeds. These are investments in your new raw food lifestyle that will reap you many rewards and steer you away from the frustration of feeling like there is "nothing to eat" when new to raw foods.

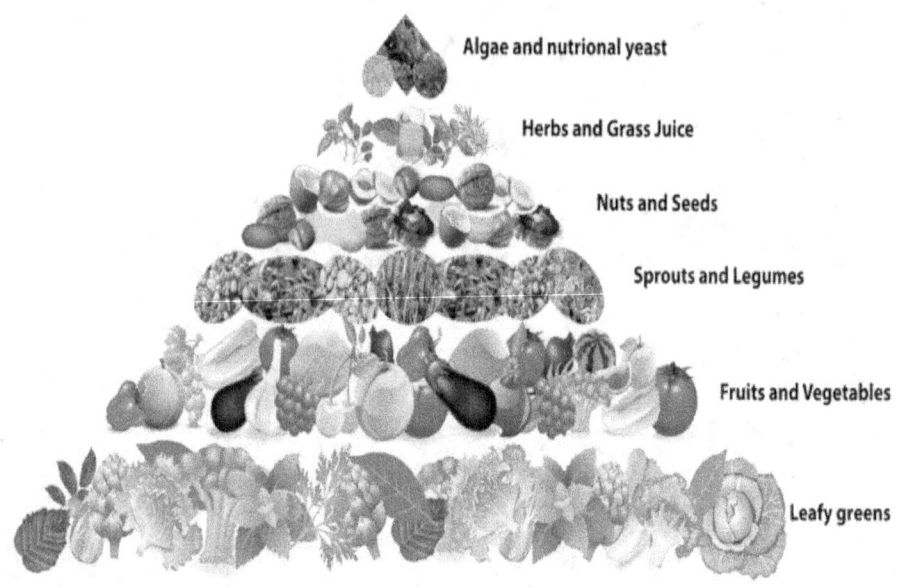

One very important point about getting started is to get a series of menu plans so you can make your food ahead f time and experiment. When getting started with raw foods, making a meal plan, even if you only loosely follow it, can relieve some of the daily pressure that can accompany a new diet and lifestyle. It saves you time at the market as well as time spent standing around the kitchen wondering what you're in the mood for. Amongst the most important nuances to plan for are new substitutions for the snacks and treats that are sprinkled throughout your days. Whether it's coffee breaks, birthday cakes, midnight snacks, or a day at the beach, you don't want to find yourself in the situation where everyone has some yummy little treat except you! So plan ahead and incorporate some of your favorite morsels into the kitchen schedule.

I found the above very helpful as I tried at first to find substitutes for the foods I most enjoyed and then started to branch out and test new recipes. Learn as much as you can about the raw vegan diet. Prepare yourself to answer some questions about nutrition, where you get your raw vegan protein, and what you eat for dinner. There may even be times when you feel that you have to defend your choices. Having all the right information at the ready will guide you through your days as you choose your meals, and it will permanently change the way you look at food.

2.6 A typical raw kitchen

This may come as a surprise to many due to so much misinformation on the Web but a raw kitchen is actually very easy to put together and can take up a lot less room than most "normal" kitchens. For starters, you do not need a microwave or a stove-top or even an oven.

A raw, vegan kitchen is the definition of simplicity. I have heard form many folks not familiar with raw preparation stating it must be difficult as your food must be prepared fresh each day. This is not the case. My wife and I prepare most of my food a couple of mornings a week for the week ahead. While we do make salads and often smoothies each day, the bulk of the food is made ahead of time, usually several days in advance. Therefore very little of our time is spent cooking or preparing food, unlike most folks. For example, I take about five minutes every three of four days to make my cashew yogurt and it will then last for days. Preparing raw food actually takes less time than cooking and therefore we have more time to do the other things we enjoy.

- **A blender** such as a Vita-mix or something comparable. If money is not too much of an issue than we highly recommend the Vitamix. We have had ours for years and have definitely put it through it's paces. Out of almost 10 years of extensive use, the only part we had to replace was the pitcher. An amazing piece of hardware.

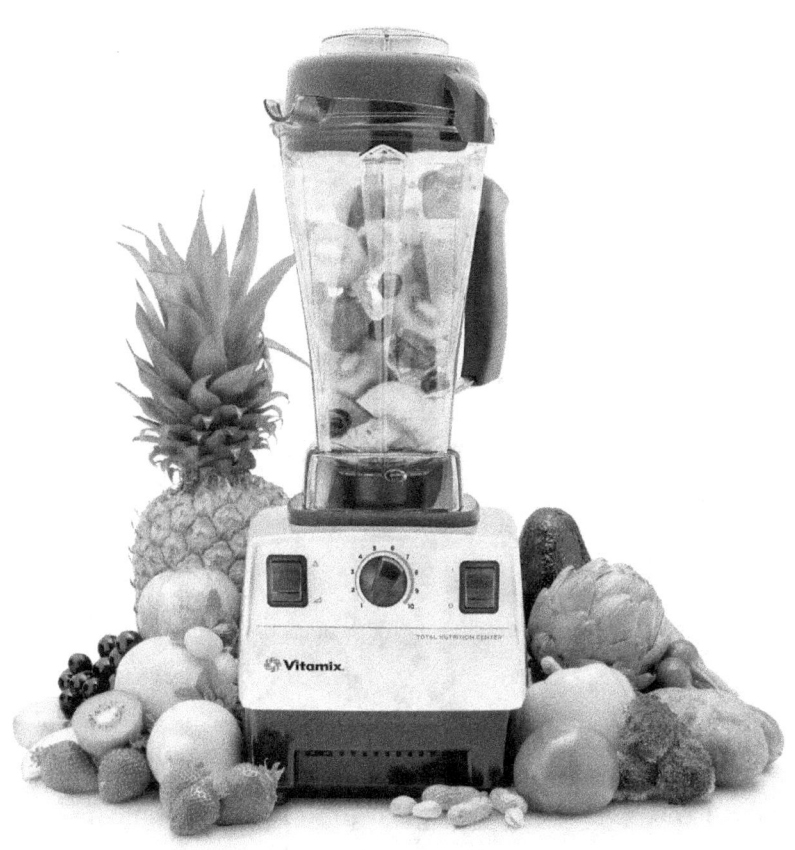

- **A Magic bullet.** What a wonderful little device. It is wonderful for quick single meals where you do not want to spend too much time in the kitchen. You can find them online or at a multitude of stores such as Walmart, Target, Costco and such.

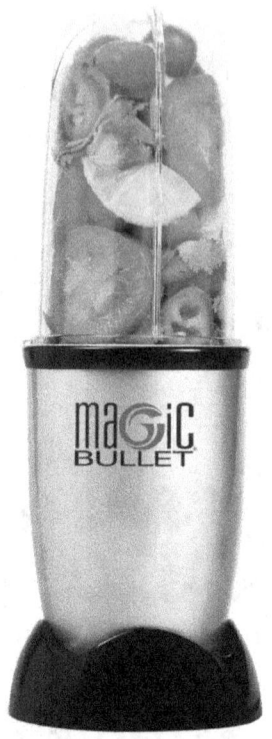

- **A food processor.** Our favorite brand is a Hamilton Beach. It is not very expensive and does a great job of chopping/dicing our veggies without turning them to mush. Also very good for chopping up nuts. Again, Target, Walmart and Costco are great sources for a food processor.

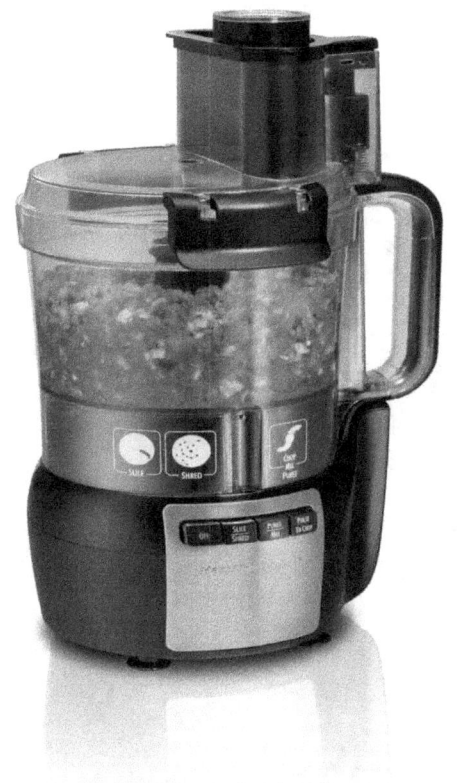

- **A juicer.** There are so many great juicers our there, some very affordable and some quite expensive. A very good mid-range cost effective juicer, the same one used in the documentary "Fat, Sick and Nearly Dead" is the Breville Juicer. It has served us well and is relatively easy to clean. But I have to say, for years we used a basic Jack Lalanne juicer, very inexpensive and it lasted through two years of very heavy use. The Breville is available at Bed, Bath and Beyond as well as in store and various other online sites. Jack Lelanne is available at Target, Walmart as well as other stores.

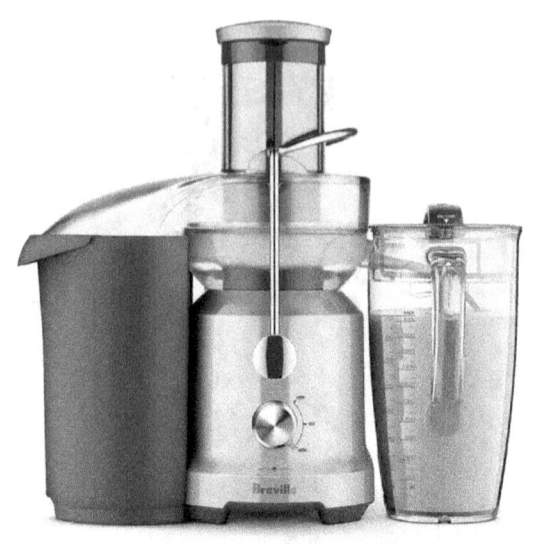

Breville Juicer

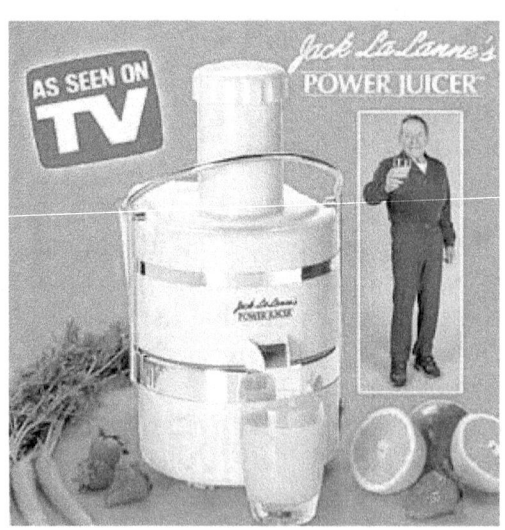

Jack Lalanne Juicer

- **A dehydrator.** This may be one of the most important pieces of equipment you can buy, especially when you are still relatively new to raw and still crave those warm, meals that can also have a crunch to them. There are many a cold Winter night I have come home to a warm raw meal or soup or lasagna my wife prepared for me. Hands down, the best dehydrator we have found in the industry is the Excalibur. While cost effective, it is also very good at its job and comes in a variety of models meant to fit your individual needs. We use the Excalibur 9 tray with a thermostat and timer. We do not use the timer very much but for raw foodist the thermostat is extremely important. We never recommend having the temperature setting above 105 degrees, in order to keep the enzymes still alive and active. A great source for the Excalibur is through Amazon online.

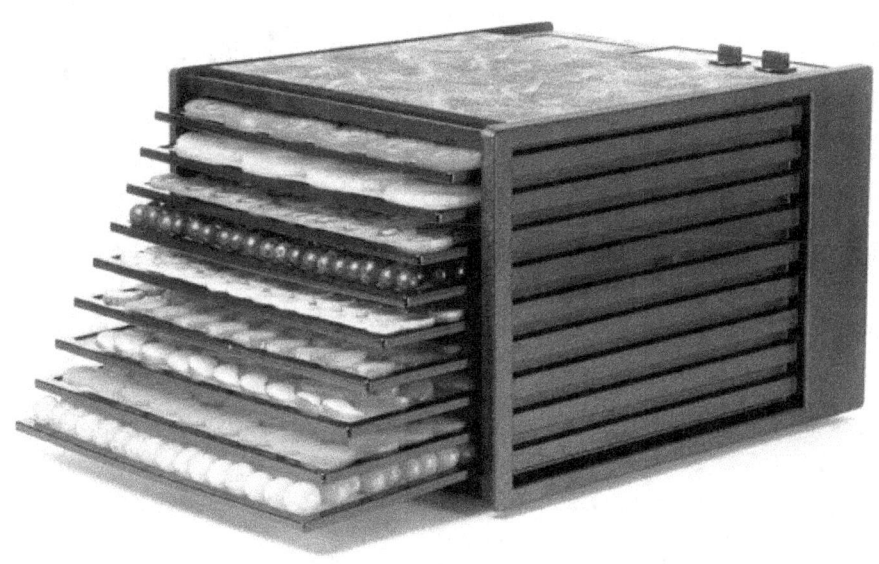

- **A nut bag.** What a simply piece of equipment and yet how valuable as a time saver. One of things we make so much of is nut milk, as well as using the left over nut meat from the process. This handy little bag allows you to easily and quickly squeeze the milk out of the bag after you have processed the milk in your blender. What's left in the bag is the meat of the nuts and we use it as well for making raw breads and such. We found them on Amazon at very reasonable prices.

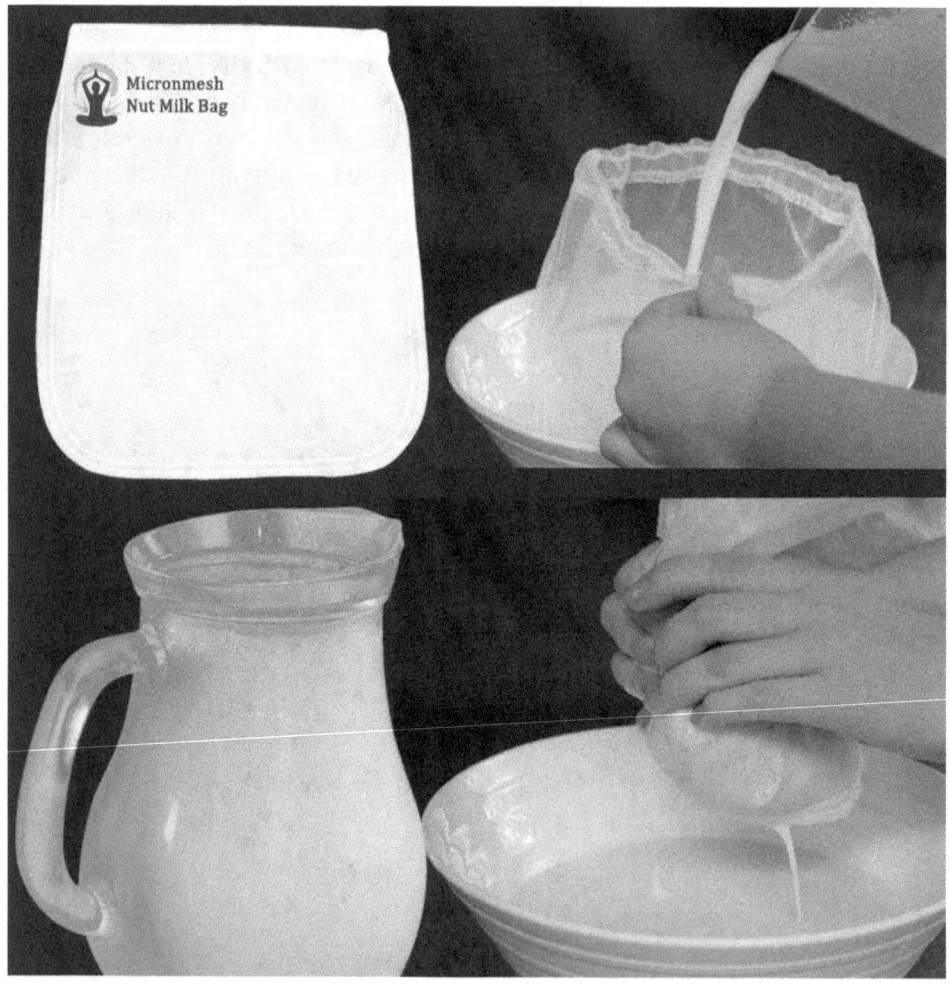

- **A sprouting jar.** So handy when you are not comfortable buying your sprouts from the grocery store. We prefer to make our own as we can make sure that only organic seeds are being used and that unhealthy city water was not used in the process. We have more control over how they were grown. And very little beats fresh sprouts from your fridge that you helped grow.

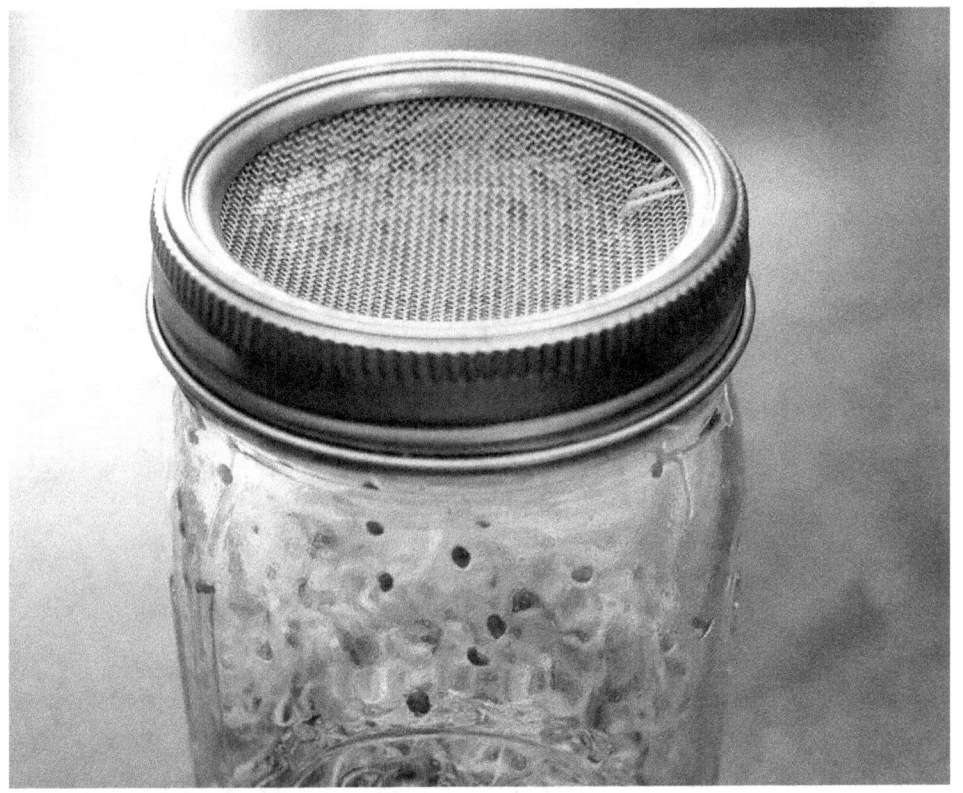

- **A wide mouth thermos.** This piece of equipment is usually not used very often but it is wonder if you are trying to make oatmeal that is still alive and full of active enzymes. It has been our practice to teach our patients the method of making oatmeal with real oat groats using the thermos method. We will be discussing this recipe later in the book. For most of our patients who try this method, very few ever go back to eating oatmeal the old, unhealthy way. Our favorite thermos is by Stanley but there are many out there. They can be fond online as well as at Walmart, Target and such.

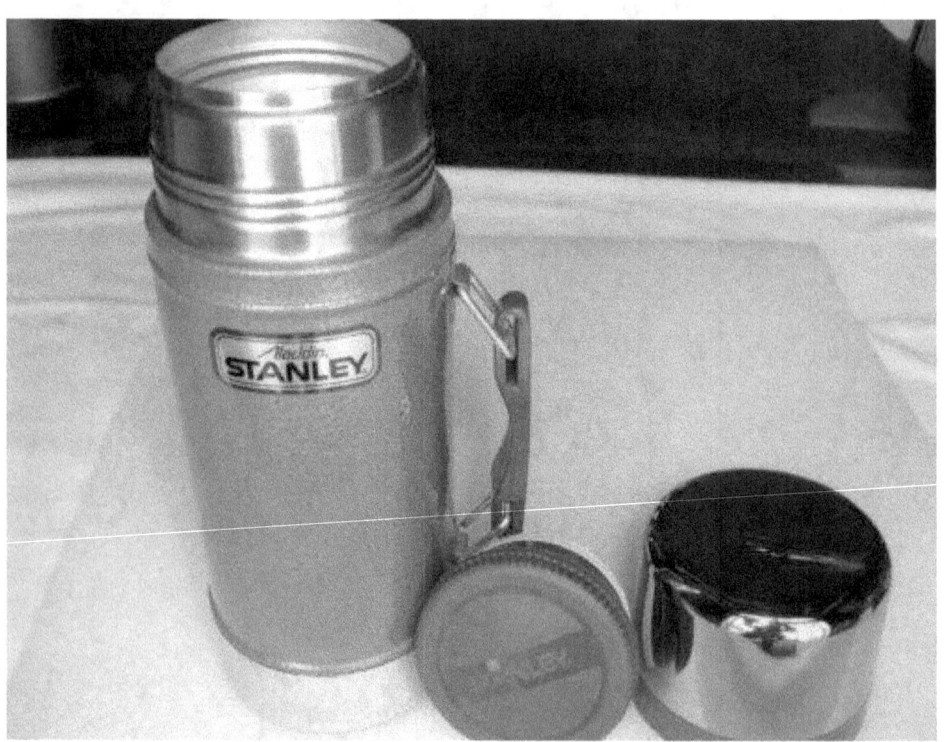

Seeds

Seed Type	Dry Measure	Soak Time	Sprout Time	Yield	Notes
Alfalfa	3 tablespoons	5 hours	5 days	4 cups	
Buckwheat	1 cup	6 hours	5-7 days	3 cups	
Clover	3 tablespoons	5 hours	5 days	4 cups	
Fenugreek	¼ cup	6 hours	5 days	4 cups	Mucous dissolving
Flax	1:1 seed/water	8 hours	-	-	Soak only
Hemp	-	-	-	-	Do not soak
Kale	¼ cup	5 hours	5 days	4 cups	
Mustard	3 tablespoons	5 hours	5 days	4 cups	
Pumpkin	1 cup	4 hours	24 hours	2 cups	Hulled
Radish	3 tablespoons	6 hours	5 days	4 cups	
Sesame	1:1 seed/water	4 hours	-	-	Hulled; Soak only
Sunflower	1 cup	4 hours	24 hours	2.5 cups	Hulled; use quickly, spoils easily

Grains

Seed Type	Dry Measure	Soak Time	Sprout Time	Yield	Notes
Amaranth	1 cup	3 hours	24 hours	3 cups	
Barley	1 cup	6 hours	5-7 days	3 cups	
Kamut	1 cup	6 hours	5-7 days	3 cups	
Millet	1 cup	3 hours	12 hours	3 cups	
Quinoa	1 cup	3 hours	24 hours	3 cups	
Rye	1 cup	6 hours	5-7 days	3 cups	
Spelt	1 cup	6 hours	5-7 days	3 cups	
Wheat	1 cup	6 hours	5-7 days	3 cups	

Nuts

Seed Type	Dry Measure	Soak Time	Sprout Time	Yield	Notes
Almonds	1 cup	12 hours	-	-	Store in refrigerator
Pecans	1 cup	1-2 hours	-	-	
Walnuts	1 cup	1-2 hours	-	-	

Beans

Seed Type	Dry Measure	Soak Time	Sprout Time	Yield	Notes
Adzuki	1 cup	8-12 hours	2-4 days	2 cups	
Garbanzo	1 cup	8-12 hours	2-3 days	2 cups	Also called chickpeas
Lentil	1 cup	8-12 hours	2-3 days	2 cups	
Mung	1 cup	8-12 hours	2-5 days	2 cups	
Peas	1 cup	8-12 hours	2-3 days	2 cups	

Length at Harvest: Sprout most seeds 1-2 inches, grains up to 4 inches, and beans ¼ to 1 inch. Exceptions include pumpkin, sunflower, amaranth, millet and quinoa which stay very short – 1/8 –1/4 inch only.

Condiments including spices, raw nuts.

A short list of some of the most widely used spices, nuts and condiment's, especially at our home:

Garlic powder

Onion powder

Himalayan pink salt

Black sea salt (amazing for egg substitutes. We will include the recipe later in this book).

Braggs Liquid Aminos (excellent as a substitute for soy sauce)

Braggs Apple Cider Vinegar

Cinnamon

Dulce and kelp, raw seaweeds such as Nori.

Dill weed

Turmeric

Nutritional yeast (What does this not go great with? Wonderful as a cheesy flavored substitute).

Mexican and Italian spices

Pumpkin spice.

Cayenne, both powdered and flakes.

Vanilla extract

Chives

Celery seeds

Ginger

Rosemary

Thyme

Sage

Curry

Paprika

Basil

Cumin

Nutmeg

All Spice

Cloves

Black pepper

Parsley

Cacao

Oregano

Coconut Oil and butter as well as dried coconut

Psyllium husk (Used as a raw thickener)

Organic, cold pressed, extra virgin Olive oil

Coconut wraps.

Raw agave

And so many more...

NUTS/SEEDS AND ASSORTED DRIED FRUITS AND VEGGIES

Cashews (You will be amazed what can be made from them)

Macadamias

Almonds

Wild jungle peanuts (actually a member of the peanut family but can be eaten raw and have no issues with fungus such as inflicting American peanuts)

Sunflower seeds

Chia seeds

Pistachios

Dates

Sun dried tomatoes

Raisins

Pepitas (pumpkin seeds)

Wild rice

Pine nuts

Walnuts

Pecans

Alfalfa and radish seeds for sprouting

Now go and explore and find more!

2.7 Beware of adulterated foods

It is sad to say that we have to be so careful about whether our food is contaminated or something clean and healing for our bodies. In a world filled with genetically modified mutations of food products, laced with chemical fertilizers, pesticides and hormones, we have to be more on guard than ever before in human history.

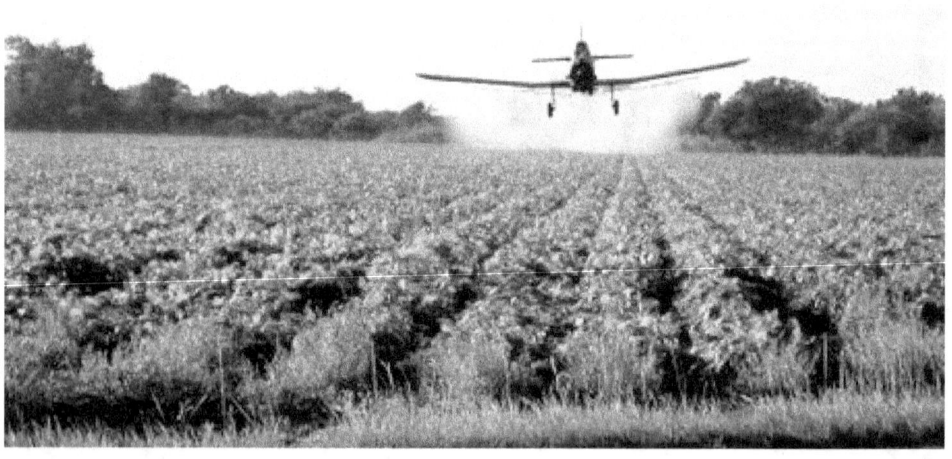

American agriculture dumps a billion pounds of pesticides on food, producing a truly toxic harvest.

According to the EPA:

- Pesticide use in agriculture is down *slightly*, from 948 million pounds in 2000 to 877 million pounds in 2007. But that's only about 1% per year, and still close to a billion pounds of toxic chemicals intentionally introduced into the environment and our food supply each year.

- Use of organophosphates continues to decline, and this definitely is a good thing, as these are among the most acutely toxic pesticides still used. But 33 million pounds is still 33 million pounds too many, and despite the decline these neurotoxins are still detected in the bodies of most Americans (see the CDC's *National Report on Human Exposure to Environmental Chemicals*) and commonly found on our food.
- The herbicide glyphosate has more than doubled in use, from 85-90 million pounds in 2001 to 180-185 million pounds in 2007. According to a report from the Organic Center, this increase is likely a reflection of the rising popularity of Monsanto's RoundUp Ready genetically modified crops. (Glyphosate is the active ingredient of RoundUp.)

In many cases, Europe is far ahead of the United States when it comes to banning certain pesticides. Here are five pesticides allowed in the U.S. but prohibited elsewhere:

1. **Neonicotinoids, or "neonics," are the main suspect in the mysterious mass disappearance of entire bee colonies** and work as nerve agents on the bees. In 2013, the European Union voted to ban three of the most common: imidacloprid, clothianidin and thiamethoxam. Those pesticides, and others in the neonic class, are still used widely in the United States, to much controversy. Despite a 2013 lawsuit from a coalition of activists and beekeepers, the EPA has said it will continue to review evidence of neonics' effects on bees until 2018.

2. **Paraquat, a pesticide linked to Parkinson's disease**, is banned in China and the European Union but not the U.S. It's highly toxic and kills weeds on contact. A 2009 UCLA study found that a person exposed to paraquat and two other pesticides is three times as likely to develop Parkinson's disease. Paraquat also can cause kidney damage and difficulty breathing. The EU voted to ban paraquat in 2007, and China approved a ban in 2012. Paraquat is famous for two things: the Drug Enforcement Administration's spraying of Mexican marijuana fields

in the 1970s, and being a leading agent of suicide in Asia and other areas.

3. **A volatile and toxic pesticide called 1,3-D (short for 1,3-Dichloropropene) is one of the most heavily used pesticides in California.** Also known as Telone, the chemical is actually a gas, or a fumigant in pesticide speak. Growers inject it into the ground to sterilize the soil before planting. But the gas evaporates easily; sometimes, it escapes from beneath its tarp and travels into nearby communities, where it poses a cancer risk to residents. The EU began phasing it out in 2007 because of its risk to humans and animals. There aren't national numbers for the U.S., but in California, the use of 1,3-D is on the rise.

4. **Glyphosate, the active ingredient in Monsanto's Roundup**, will soon to be banned in the Netherlands Brazil is considering a ban. Ontario, Canada, banned it for home use as a "cosmetic" pesticide (chemicals that keep your yard looking nice). This year, Sri Lanka banned it. Scientists suspect it may be the culprit in widespread kidney disease among agricultural workers in Sri Lanka, India and Central America. It's the best-selling herbicide in the world, according to the Ag Journal. And it was the most heavily used pesticide in the U.S. in 2007, according to the most recent number available from the EPA.

5. **A popular herbicide called atrazine is the pesticide most commonly found in American drinking water.** The European Union banned it in 2004 but the EPA re-evaluated and OK'd atrazine use in 2009. While it breaks down quickly in soil, it tends to hang around in water. Almost 90 percent of drinking water in the U.S. has atrazine in it, according to an analysis of U.S. Department of Agriculture data by the Pesticide Action Network. The weed killer messes with hormones, affects the immune system and is linked to birth defects. A New York Times investigation in 2009 found that levels of atrazine in some communities' drinking water have spiked, sometimes for longer than a month. Residents were not told, mainly because local water authorities didn't know about the pesticide. Forty-three water authorities that did know sued atrazine's manufacturer, Syngenta.

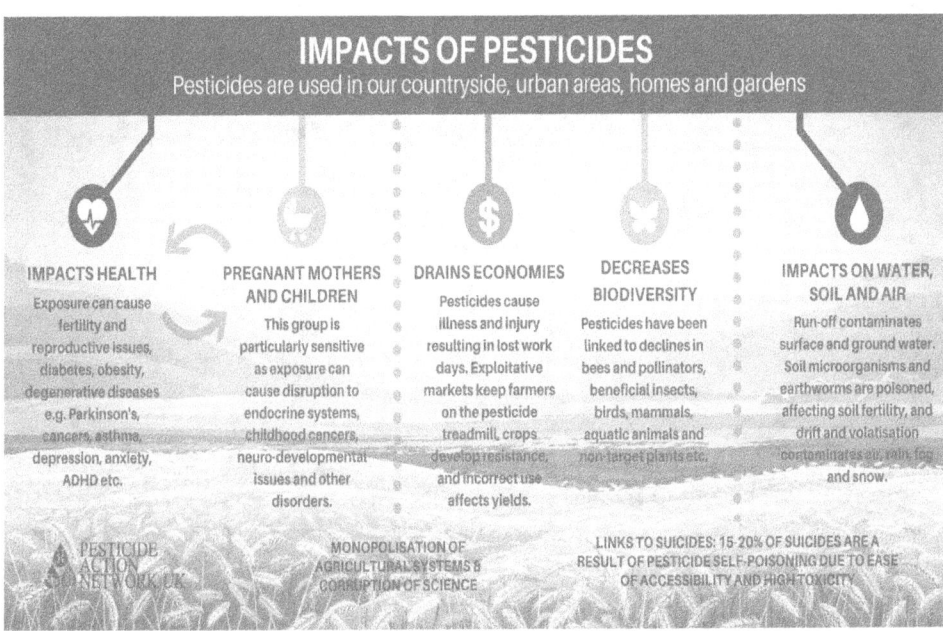

When it comes to finding healthy, organic produce it becomes yet another difficult proposition. Only 1% of crops in America to date are certified organic. Why? It is not due to low demand. It is in the regulation red tape. It takes a farmer three years of growing without chemicals before they are allowed to call their produce organic. So unfortunately, most of the organic crops are being shipped in from other countries. This means the majority of crops grown in America are either laced with extensive chemicals and/or are GMO (genetically modified organisms).

In 2019, 94 percent of the soybean crops in the United States were genetically modified to be herbicide tolerant. Genetically modified crops have taken agriculture in the U.S. by storm. By comparison, only 17 percent of soybean crops were genetically modified in 1997. Other crops grown in the United States which are mostly genetically modified are cotton and corn. Currently, 65% of produce samples analyzed by the U.S. Department of Agriculture test positive for pesticide residues? Unless you're buying certified organic food, the chances are that you're consuming a significant amount of chemicals with every portion of your 'healthy' greens.

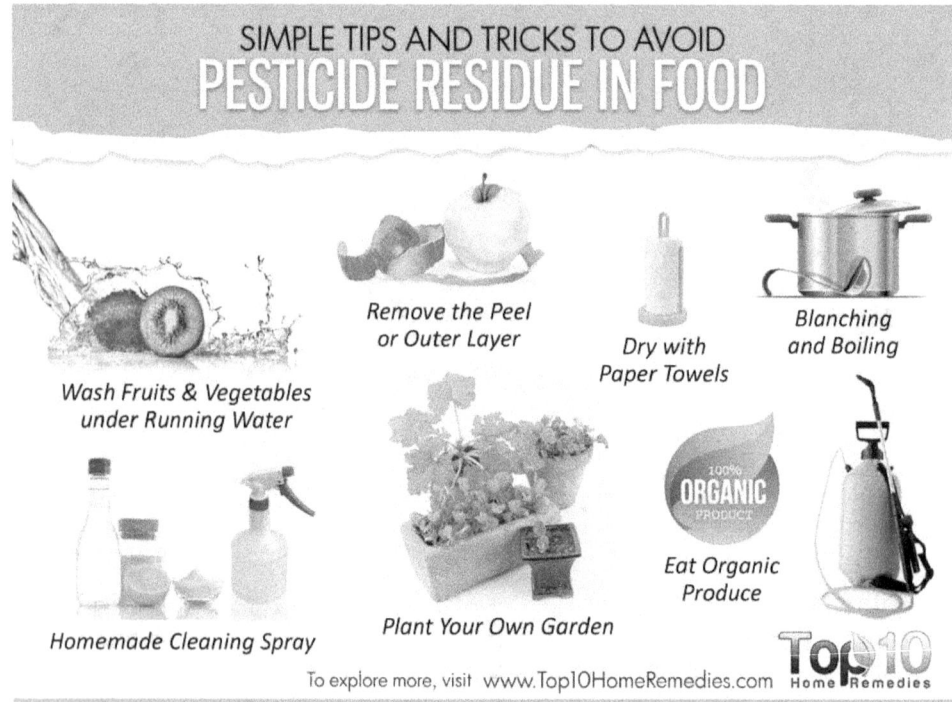

So, what can we do? For one trick you can simply wash your fresh produce in distilled white vinegar and water solution. And of course, as the picture above shows, buy as much organic as you can.

CHAPTER 3

RECIPES

3.1 Breakfast

OAT MEAL IN A THERMOS

Now.. there is a way to get some oats in a safe and very tasty manner. I am going to include a method here for making oatmeal which is still VERY high in enzymes, vitamins, minerals and produces an alkaline reaction. Here ya go:

You will need:
1.) Oat Groats. You can get them at the health food store and grain stores. Make SURE they are OAT GROATS and organic if you can, not steel cut, nothing else.
2.) Water, preferred distilled of course.
3.) A good thermos.

We usually do this about 7:00 or so in the evening prior to the morning that we would like them for breakfast.

OK, pour oat groats into thermos until it is 1/4 to 1/3 full of them.
Boil the water and then pour into thermos until about an inch of air space is left at the top. This is so the oat groats can expand over night.
Close tight the thermos and shake well. Then place in corner of kitchen until morning.
In the morning pop the top and the oats should still be nice and warm and smelling wonderful!

You can use raw almond milk with them along with organic agave, bananas, raisins, apples, etc. This is how I have my oatmeal.

RAW ALMOND MILK

As for the raw almond milk being expensive to make, here is how I do it very cheaply:

1 cup raw almond soaked for 4 hours or more (I do overnight).
4 cups filtered or distilled water.
1/4 cup agave
Pinch of salt
A few drops of vanilla (optional)

In a high speed blender or a vita mix blend nuts and water for about two minutes.
Then filter through a double cheesecloth, cotton diaper or the milk bag. Save the meat for breads and other things.
Put milk back into blender and add the other ingredients and blend again.
AWESOME!

Oat Meal #2

Serves 2

Ingredients:
2 apples
1 banana
1 tablespoon golden flax seed
2 teaspoons cinnamon
Pure water

Directions:
Put the flax seeds in the purified water and let sit overnight.
Peel the apples and cut them in smaller parts (for the blender). Peel the banana and break in parts. Rinse the flax seeds.
Put all ingredients in a blender. This can be a hand blender or high speed blender such as Vitamix. Add 1/4 cup water, just enough to let the mixture blend well. Blend all ingredients until smooth. You may want to add a little more water if it's too thick.

Tip
You make this recipe even better by replacing the water with almond milk or fresh juice. You may also add a tablespoon of hemp seeds. You can also add (germinated) nuts and raisins. You can prepare this recipe the night before (but put the banana in there in the morning). Especially with nuts and dried fruits in it, it will only taste better!
 I like this breakfast because it has healthy ingredients that are easy to get: especially, the fiber, good fats and protein of the flax seeds.

Hemp & Berry Smoothie

Serves 2

Ingredients:
1 banana
2 tablespoons hulled hemp seed
1 bag of frozen berries
1 cup pure water

Directions:
Put all ingredients in a high speed blender. Add enough water so that all ingredients are covered. Blend well.
You may want to add a little more water if it's too thick. You may blend longer if you find it too cold.

Tip
This is such a yummy and easy breakfast recipe.
The hemp seeds provide good fats and super protein. Hemp seeds are the only seeds that have no enzyme inhibitor and therefore don't have to be soaked in water before eating.
If the berries are sour, you may add a few drops of (liquid) stevia or agave to sweeten.

Carrot Juice

Serves 1

Ingredients:
2 pounds carrots
1/2 lemon

Directions:
Wash the lemon and cut most of the peel off. Juice the lemon and the carrots.
Ready!
Tip

If I take this juice for breakfast, I feel so good the rest of the day. It gives me instant energy.
I also like to juice about a 1/2 bunch green leafy vegetables with the carrots for extra alkalizing minerals. Carrot greens, kale or lettuce are a good choice. Apples, celery and fennel also go well with carrot juice. If you're a beginner, start to add only one or two leafs of greens to make sure you still like it. Greens are an acquired taste and it may take some time for you to get use to.

Young Coconut Water

Serves 1

Ingredients:
1 young coconut

Directions:
Open the coconut with a cleaver. Talking about easy, quick and healthy!

Tip
You may pour the water in the jar of a high speed blender and some or all of the milk. Blend and you get yourself coconut milk. You can also pour some of the milk into ice cubes - it freezes really easily - and whenever you make a smoothie you can add some coconut milk ice cube for an even more delicious smoothie. Especially quick for breakfast.

Green Drink

Serves 1

Ingredients:
1 scoop green powder
16 ounce pure water

Directions:
Add one scoop to the water and mix. Ready!

Tip
You can put this in a water bottle and take with you. If you don't like the taste of the green powder, you may add some lemon juice or add to another juice.

Banana Pancakes

Serves 1

Ingredients:
1 banana
2 tablespoons coconut meal or dried coconut flakes
cinnamon

Directions:
Mash the banana with a fork in a bowl until very smooth. Add the coconut meal and some cinnamon to taste. Mix well.

Flatten the banana/coconut dough and make small pancakes of them. Leave out in direct sunlight for about 1 hour, flip over and leave for another hour. You may also use the dehydrator or oven. But then it will take longer to dry them.

They don't have to be dry, just on the outsides. They're so good anyway that they're usually gone before I want to serve them.

Tip
If you make them the night before, you can take them to go for breakfast in the morning.

Granola

Serves 1

Ingredients:
Raw Granola
Vanilla raw yogurt (see next recipe)

Directions:
In the US you can buy raw granola at most health food stores. You may eat this with vanilla yogurt (see recipe below), almond milk or apple avocado mouse. Another yummy breakfast recipe.

Vanilla raw yogurt

Serves 1

Ingredients:
1/2 cup coconut water
1 cup coconut meat
1/2 teaspoon vanilla extract

Directions:

Open the coconut with a cleaver. Pour the coconut water in the jar of a high speed blender and some or all of the milk. Blend well. You should get the consistency of yogurt.

Tip

You can drink it as is or you can add a fruit of your choice. Think of peach, strawberries, mango or pear. So good! A fantastic replacer of yogurt made from dairy. It's delicious as a yogurt desert, for breakfast with granola or you can put in in your ice maker machine and you get delicious ice cream.

Apple Avocado Mousse

Serves 2

Ingredients:
1 avocado
2 apples
1/4 cup purified water

Directions:
Peal the apples and take out the core. Take the avocado meat out of the avocado. Put the two ingredients in a bowl. Mix well with a hand mixer.

RAW BREAKFAST CREPES

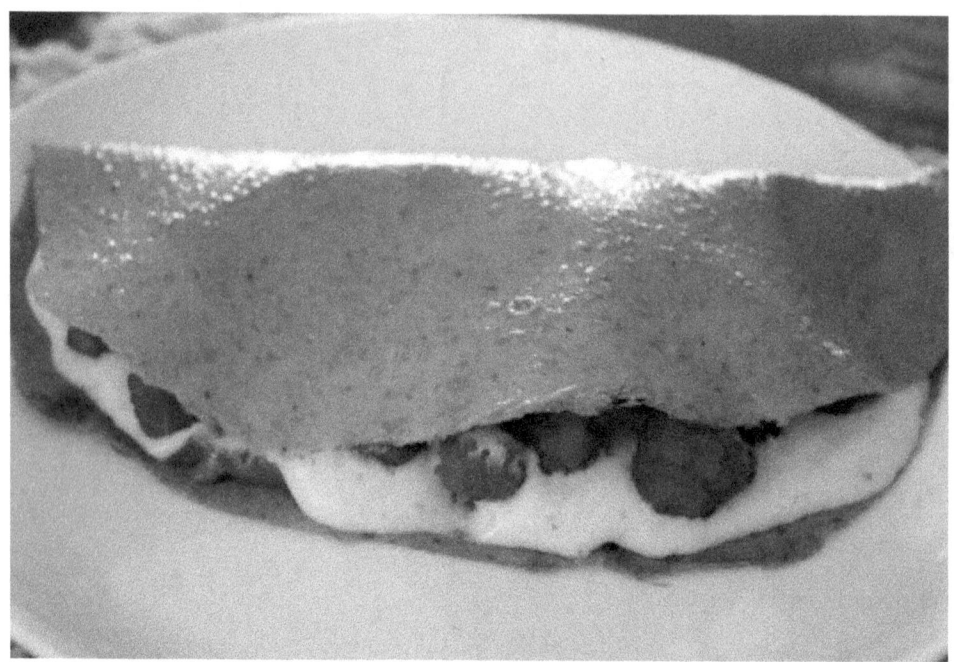

Description:
The weekend is upon us and we highly recommend whipping up something decadent yet healthy for brunch tomorrow morning - you deserve it! These are Gena Hemshaw's simple raw vegan crepes with a banana soft serve filling and fresh strawberry jam. Gooey, chewy, and totally delish!

Cuisine Phase 2 Makes 2 crepes

For the crepes:
2 large or 3 small ripe bananas
1 teaspoon ground flax seed

For the Strawberry "Jam" (NB: this technique was one of my favorite discoveries from my homegirl Sarma's Raw Food, Real World. She's a genius, that one!)

1 cup sliced strawberries

For the Cream Layer:
1 batch banana soft serve

For the filling:
1/2 cup berries of choice

Methods/steps For the crepes:

1) Place the bananas and flax in a food processor. Process until the mix is a very smooth liquid.

2) Line two dehydrator sheets with teflex. Pour half of the liquid onto one of them and spread it with a spatula or inverted spatula. You want to aim for it to be relatively thin (let's say 1/8 inch). Smooth it into a circular shape; this can be messy, since you'll make the edges pretty later on. Repeat with the other half of the banana mix on another sheet. Dehydrate at 115 degrees for 3 hours, or until the crepes are totally smooth to the touch (careful, if you check these before they're ready, you'll likely mess up the surface! Think of this as drying nail polish: don't touch it till you're pretty sure it's hard enough.)

3) When the crepes are truly ready, remove them from the dehydrator, and very CAREFULLY peel the crepe from the teflex sheet. Trace a perfect circle on the crepe (I used the lid of a pot to do this), and then, using a very sharp paring knife, cut a neat circle out. What's left will resemble this: For the Strawberry "Jam"

1) Place strawberries on mesh lined dehydrator sheets and dehydrate for six hours or so. When they're ready, they ought to be shrunken and dry, but clearly still a little plump inside. 2) Transfer strawberries to a food processor fitted with the "S" blade, and process till the mix resembles a messy, textured jam.

To Assemble:
1) lay out a single crepe and top with 1-2 tbsp of the jam.
2) Over that, spread 1/3 cup banana soft serve.

3) Finally, top this with 1/2 cup fresh berries.

Fold, and serve!

Banana Peach Soup

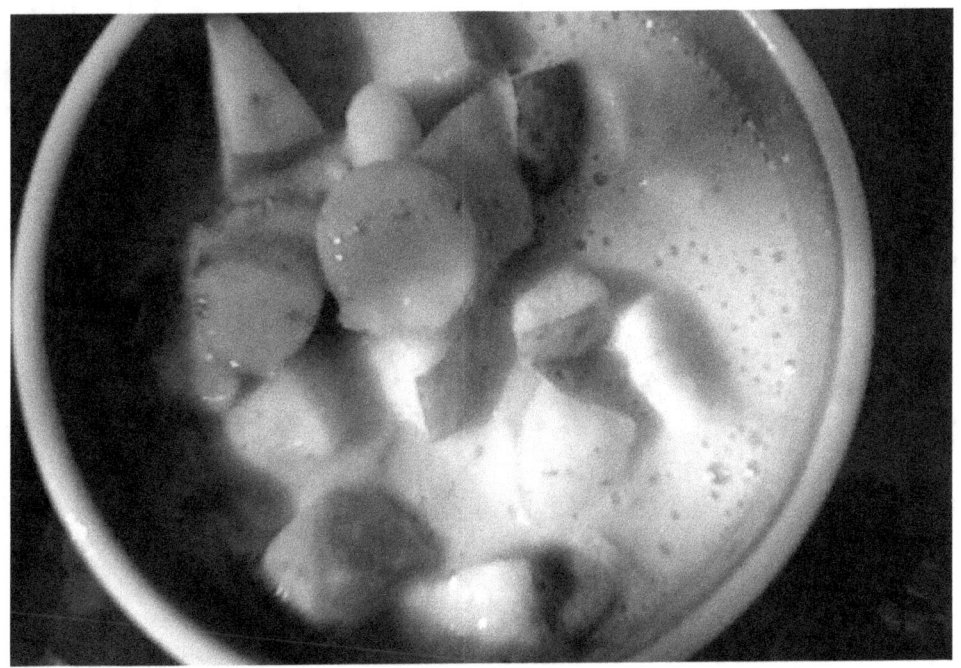

Preparation Time: 5 minutes
Servings: 1

Ingredients:
3 bananas
2 white peaches
2 yellow peaches
1 cup water

Directions:
1) Blend 2 bananas with 1 yellow and 1 white peach with some water. Slice 1 banana and 1 yellow and 1 white peach into chunks. Put the sliced fruit in a bowl and pour the blended fruit on top.
Super easy, healthy and delish! Enjoy!

RAW WAFFLES

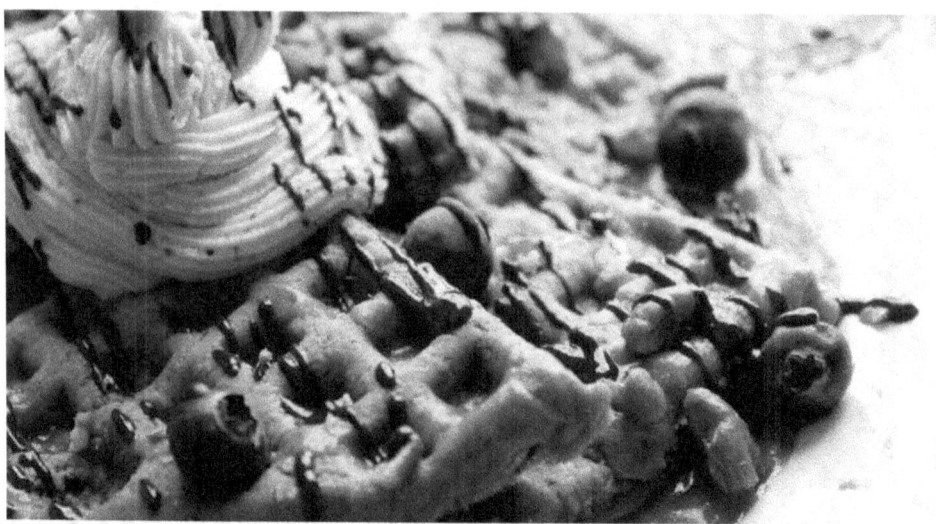

Description:
Raw waffles?! This is a truly masterful recipe, decadent yes, but also surprisingly easy to make. If you've ever wondered if it's possible to make raw vegan waffles the answer is most definitely, and with this recipe now is your chance to shine! The waffle base is a simple mixture of freshly ground flax, pecans, and soaked buckwheat groats. A perfect fusion of decadence and healthy nutrition!

Equipment Needed:
Blender Juicer
Dehydrator
Rainbow Green Cuisine
Phase 2 Makes 6 large or 12 small waffles

Waffle Batter:
1 ½ Cups flax powder
1 ½ Cups of pecans (on nut of your choice)
3 Cups soaked buckwheat
Caramel Sauce Topping:
8 tablespoons cashews or macadamia butter

2 tablespoons coconut butter
4 tablespoons coconut water- room temperature
2 tablespoons yacon syrup
2 tablespoons agave syrup
pinch of vanilla bean
1/4 teaspoon salt to a blender.

*To spice up this recipe you can add cacao nibs or chopped nuts. For example turn the caramel sauce into a turtle caramel sauce by adding cacao nibs and chopped pecans.

Dark Dipping Chocolate (chocolate sauce):
1 Cup cacao butter
1 Cup cacao powder
2 Tablespoons lucuma pinch vanilla bean
1/2 cup clear agave or sweetener of choice.
*Optional- superfood powders 1 Tablespoon collectively.

Methods/steps Waffle Batter:
1) Mix ingredients in a big mixing bowl. Affix your blank plate attachment to your twin gear masticating juicer (I like the Green Star Champion Juicer) and feed mixture through the juicer, creating the dough.

2) Take a waffle maker and cover the bottom with plastic wrap.

3) Spoon in a bit of dough and spread it evenly with your hands, making sure it covers the entire waffle iron. Making sure not to pile it too thick or spread it too thin.

4) Lay a piece of plastic wrap across the top side of your waffle and press the 2 sides of the waffle iron together firmly to achieve a nice waffle pattern on both sides. Using the plastic wrap, lift the waffle out of the waffle iron and lay bottom side up on a dehydrator tray. Trim off any unclean edges with a butter knife.

5) Dehydrate for 8 hours at 110 degrees.

6) Pull waffles out and top them as you please- fruit, chocolate sauce, caramel sauce (instructions below), wild jungle peanut butter or a combination.

Caramel Sauce Topping:
1) Blend ingredients until smooth

Dark Dipping Chocolate (chocolate sauce):
1) Using a low heat source, melt the cacao butter, preferably in a glass bowl. At the same time, place your sweetener in a dish and heat that up as well. I prefer to use my dehydrator for this.

2) Sift all powders in the melted cacao butter (This includes any superfood powders you may want to add.) and whisk together.

3) Place cacao butter/powder mixture back into the dehydrator for 5-10 minutes.

4) Take heated cacao mixture and add the heated sweetener. Whisk vigorously.

5) After the mixture is thoroughly combined, you have a chocolate that is ready to use for dipping or drizzling.

APPLE CINNAMON CREPES

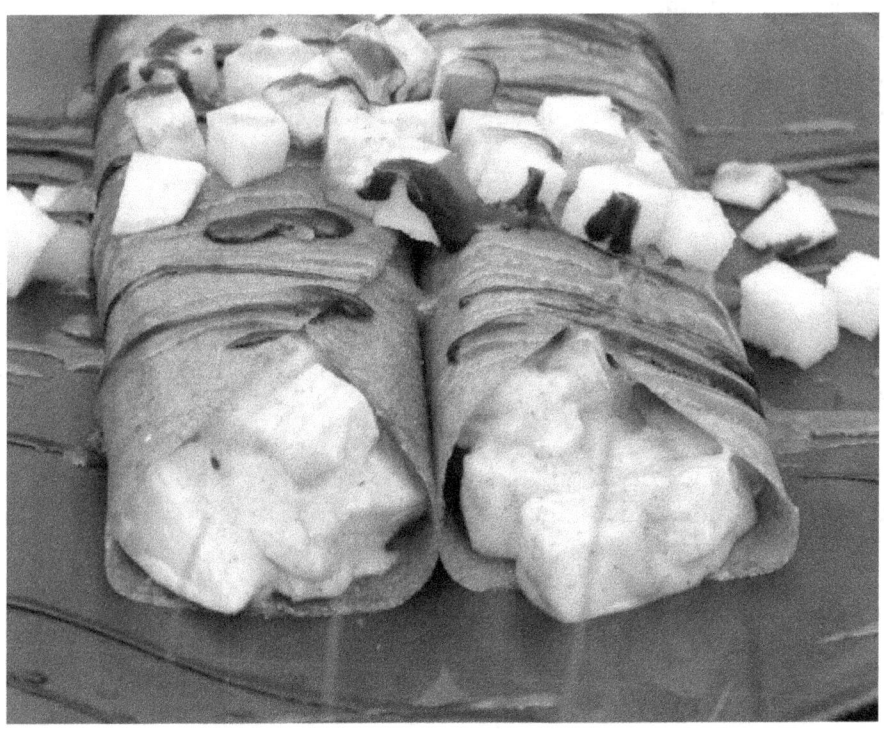

Description
Brunch is served! A gorgeous recipe for yummy banana-pear crepes with a creamy cashew and spiced apple filling. Check out Heather's Just Desserts ebook for more Sweetly Raw recipes including the chocolate and caramel sauce she's drizzled over her crepes in the photo.

Makes 4 crepes

Banana Pear Crepes:
2-3 bananas
1-2 pears Apple

Cinnamon Cream Filling:
3/4 cup cashews
5 tablespoons water

3 tablespoons Agave syrup
1/2 teaspoon cinnamon
1/2 teaspoon vanilla
Pinch of salt 1 tablespoon melted coconut oil
2-3 medium apples or pears, diced small (peeled optional)

Methods/steps

Banana Pear Crepes:
1) Blend the bananas and pears in a blender until completely smooth.

2) Pour a thin layer onto teflex dehydrator sheets and spread evenly using an offset spatula.

3) Dehydrate at 115F for 6-8 hours, or until you can peel it off the teflex. If still a little too moist/wet on the underside, continue drying for 1/2 - 1 hour. The crepe sheet should be pliable.

4) Cut the sheet into 4 squares.

Apple Cinnamon Cream Filling:

1) Blend all but the apple in a high speed blender until smooth. Set aside.

2) Fold the cream with the apples or pears - if you want a creamier filling fold in less apples and vice versa.

Assembly:

1) Spoon some apple cinnamon filling onto a crepe (If you want a more rolled up crepe, spoon a smaller amount of filling. If you want a fuller crepe, add more filling).

2) Either roll or fold over the crepe flaps. Optional: Drizzle some caramel sauce and/or chocolate sauce on top. Garnish with extra chopped apple or pear.

RAW DANISH PASTRY

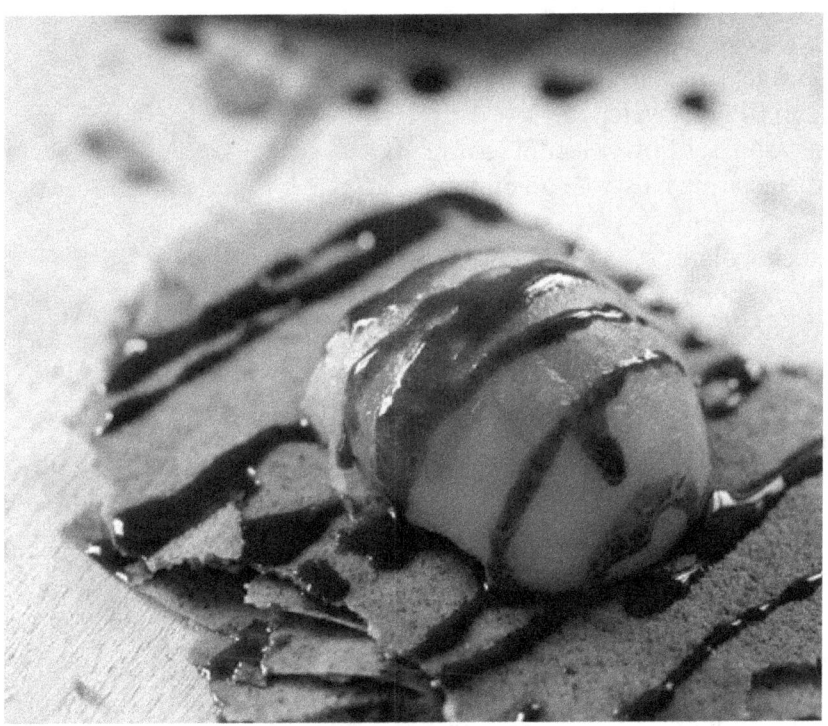

Description
A creative and truly gourmet raw vegan recipe inspired by Danish pastries, served with homemade chocolate sauce and fresh juicy nectarines! Enjoy it for your next weekend brunch!

Serves 3-4

Irish Moss Gel:
90 g soaked, rinsed Irish moss (make sure to squeeze out the water before measuring).
0.5 cup filtered Water

Remaining Ingredients for Pastry Dough:
1 cup Macadamia nuts
1 cup shredded Coconut
1.5 teaspoon real Vanilla

5 tablespoons Lúcuma (can be substituted to Mesquite)
1/4 teaspoon Himalayan salt
1.5 tablespoon juice from an organic Lemon
0.5 cup Agave nectar
1 1/4 cup filtered Water
0.5 teaspoon Sunflower lecitin (optional)
Peeled Nectarine halves to go on top.

Melted chocolate:
50 g Cacao butter (1/4 cup as melted)
2 tablespoons raw Cacao powder
2 tablespoons Agave nectar

Methods/steps

Irish Moss Gel:
1) First, make some Irish moss paste by doing the following: Soak about a cup dry irish moss in water until it softens completely. Then go through piece by piece under running water to remove any impurity (small pieces of plastic, sea shells etc.)

2) Put the irish moss in a plastic container with lid and add water, about 2/3 of the container. Put on the lid and shake the container intensely for 30 sec. Change the water and repeat two more times. As you will see the water gets cleaner and cleaner after each time. Don't rinse the irish moss too much though, as it will also wash away the carageenan (a natural gelatine) and the irish moss will not have the desired effect which is to act as a thickening agency. Don't worry about the fishy smell of the irish moss. You won't feel it once you mix it up with the rest of the ingredients!

3) Let the cleaned irish moss soak in water for 3-4 hours for it to swell further.

4) Use a scissor to cut the irish moss into pieces and put it in a high speed blender together with 0.5 cup filtered water and blend until smooth. This will take some time and you will want to work with a spatula to scrape down any bits of irish moss from the inside of the lid and jar of your blender. Your

blender is going to heat up from all the blending, so that the irish moss paste become lukewarm. That is good as it activates the carageenan.

5) Transfer the ready made irish moss paste to a little bowl / cup. It should be thick and smooth, not watery. The first time you do this it might seem complicated, but it really isn't. Continue with the rest of the ingredients for the paper thin pastry dough:

Remaining Ingredients for Pastry Dough:
1) Grind the Macadamia nuts and shredded Coconut in a high speed blender into a fine flour.

2) Add the rest of the dry ingredients and mix well.

3) Now add the Irish moss gel, Lemon juice, Agave, Water and Sunflower lecitin and process until completely smooth.

4) Pour the mixture over a dehydrator mesh screen with a plastic sheet on top. It is important that the mixture is as thin as possible. The technique you use to succeed with that is that you start pouring about a cup of the mixture over the sheet. Then you lean the mesh screen to one side, letting the mixture slide down. Do this in all four directions until the mixture is evenly spread. Also work with a spatula. When it is as thin as possible, you carefully shake it sideways to create a perfectly even surface, just like you would do when swirling two batters for a raw cheesecake *you will see what I mean*.

5) Do this with two more mesh screens and put them into the dehydrator and start drying them in 105 F. Flipping Time: After 12 hours, you can flip the paper thin pastry dough, by putting a mesh net on top of the pastry, hold it firmly with your palms and flip it carefully. Then you remove the mesh net that's been under the downside of the pastry dough, and peel off the mesh sheet by pulling in one corner. It's all quite logic. Continue to dry the pastry dough for another 7-8 hours and you are done. Total Drying Time: 19-20 hours.

Melted chocolate:

1) In a water bath or by using the dehydrator, melt the Cacao butter slowly. Then blend by using a whisk, with the Cacao powder and Agave nectar until incorporated.

2) Pour in a squeeze bottle if you have one. Otherwise you can drizzle the melted chocolate with a spoon.

Assembly:
1) Assemble the dessert by breaking off pieces in the size of your palm and put them in layers to create height. On top of them you put a ripe, halved and peeled nectarine, then drizzle the melted chocolate over it all.

CALIFORNIA ROLLS

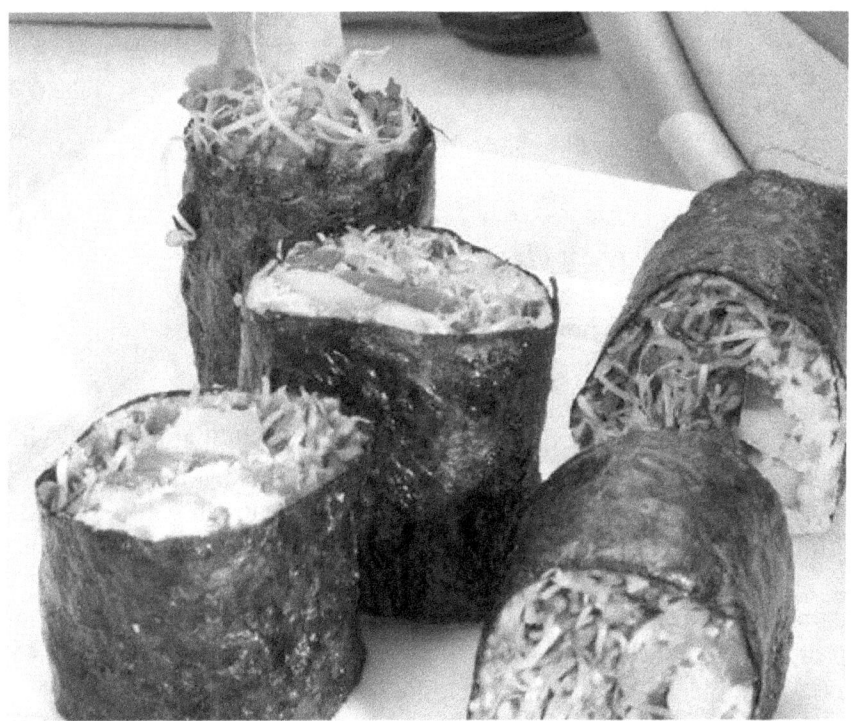

Description
California rolls are always a great option when you're craving something light, fresh, and savory! It takes a bit of practice getting your rolling technique down but once you do you'll be making sushi like a master! Follow the instructions below from Jennifer Cornbleet to create the perfect raw vegan sushi roll complete with lots of sprouts, avocado, and thinly sliced vegetables. This recipe doesn't call for any rice or sticky spread, instead it relies on a small amount of mellow white miso for added flavor and to help the nori bind together to form a roll. Taste the freshness!

Makes 2 rolls 2 nori sheets
2 teaspoons mellow white miso
2 cups alfalfa or clover sprouts (optional)
½ ripe avocado, thinly sliced
¼ cucumber, seeded and cut lengthwise into thin strips
¼ cup grated carrot

¼ red bell pepper, cut lengthwise into thin strips
Tamari for dipping (optional)

Methods/steps:

1) Lay one sheet of nori, shiny side down, on a bamboo sushi mat.

2) Using the back of a teaspoon, spread 1 teaspoon of the miso in a single horizontal strip anywhere along the bottom third of the nori.

3) Along the edge of the nori closest to you, layer half of the optional sprouts, avocado, cucumber, carrot, and bell pepper.

4) To roll, grip the edges of the nori sheet and the sushi mat together with your thumbs and forefingers, and press the filling back toward you with your other fingers. Using the mat to help you, roll the front edge of the nori over the filling. Squeeze it with the mat; then lift the mat and continue rolling.

5) Just before completing the roll, dip your index finger in water and run it along the far edge of the nori sheet. This will seal the seam of the roll. Cut the roll into 6 pieces with a serrated knife.

6) Fill, roll, and slice the other sheet of nori the same way. Arrange on a plate and serve immediately, with a small bowl of tamari for dipping, if desired.

Blood Building Beetroot, Raspberry and Vanilla Smoothie Bowl

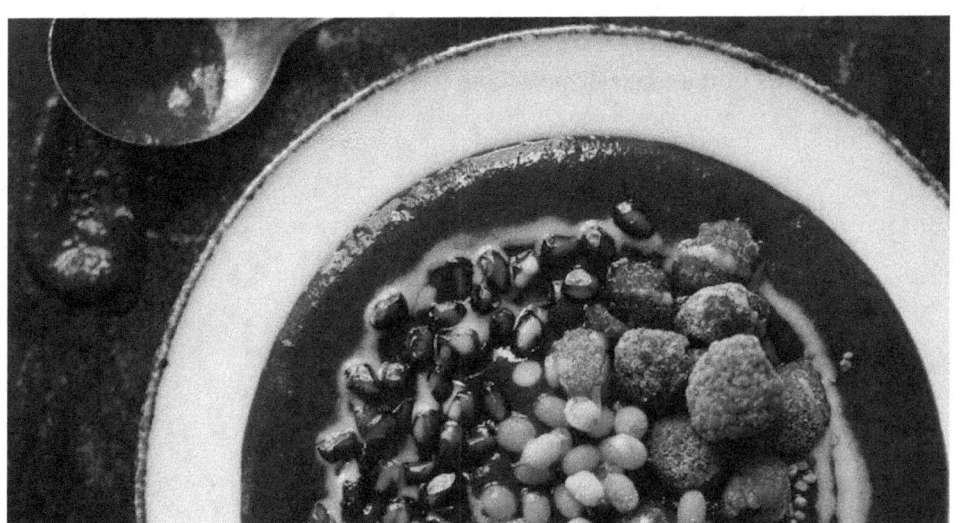

Ingredients:
- 1 small beet, peeled and chopped
- 1 cup raspberries, fresh or frozen
- 2 cups packed spinach
- 3 prunes, soaked in 1/2 cup water small wedge organic lemon (including the peel!)
- 1-2 scoops plant based protein
- 1-2 tsp. wheatgrass powder (or spirulina / chlorella) a generous pinch ground vanilla powder (or 1 tsp. vanilla extract)
- 1/2 cup water or plant based raw milk of choice
- frozen raspberries
- pomegranate seeds
- sea buckthorn berries
- bee pollen • raw almond butter

Instructions:
1. Soak prunes overnight in water, or for a minimum of one hour.

2. Pour the soaked prunes and their liquid into a blender. Add all remaining ingredients and blend on high until completely smooth (if you do not have a

high-speed blender, this may take a minute or so). Taste and adjust sweetness / vanilla / lemon as desired.

3. Pour contents into a glass or bowl and garnish with desired toppings. Enjoy!

Blueberry Bowl

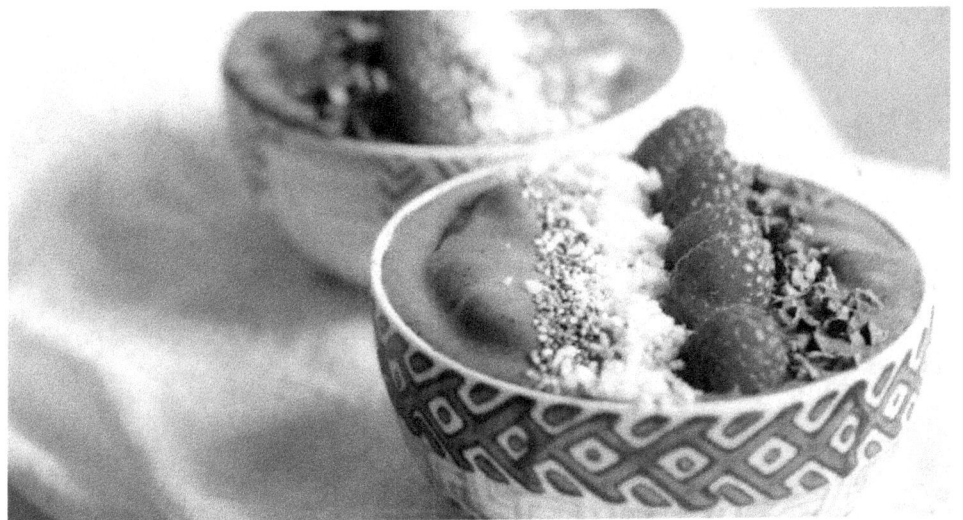

Ingredients:
- 1 cup frozen blueberries
- 1½ frozen bananas • 3/4 coconut water
- 1 tsp. vanilla extract
- 2 tsp. Maca powder(or other superfood(s) of your choice)
- Optional toppings: chia seeds, nuts, raw cacao nibs, shredded coconut, berries, banana slices, hemp seeds, goji berries, etc.

Instructions:
Add everything to your blender and blend on high until smooth and creamy. Divide between two bowls and top with all the good stuff - go crazy!

Chocolate Cherry Bomb Smoothie

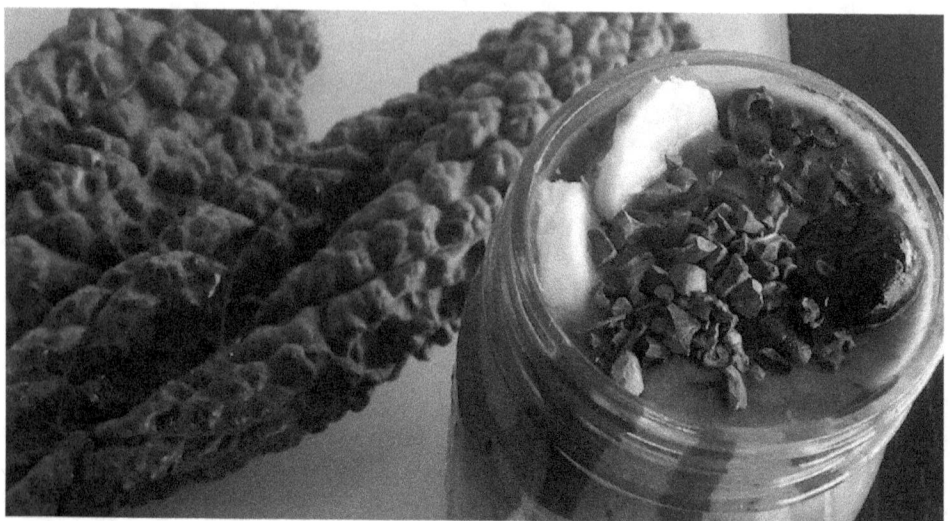

Ingredients:
- 3 stalks celery
- 2 handfuls of kale leaves
- 1 ripe banana • 1 cup of cherries
- 1-2 Tbsp cacao powder
- 1 cup of hemp (or almond) milk

Instructions:
1. Place all ingredients in a high speed blender and blend until smooth.
2. Topping: hemp seeds, goji berries, banana slices and cherries thawed overnight.

You can use frozen cherries for thicker consistency.

Frappaccino

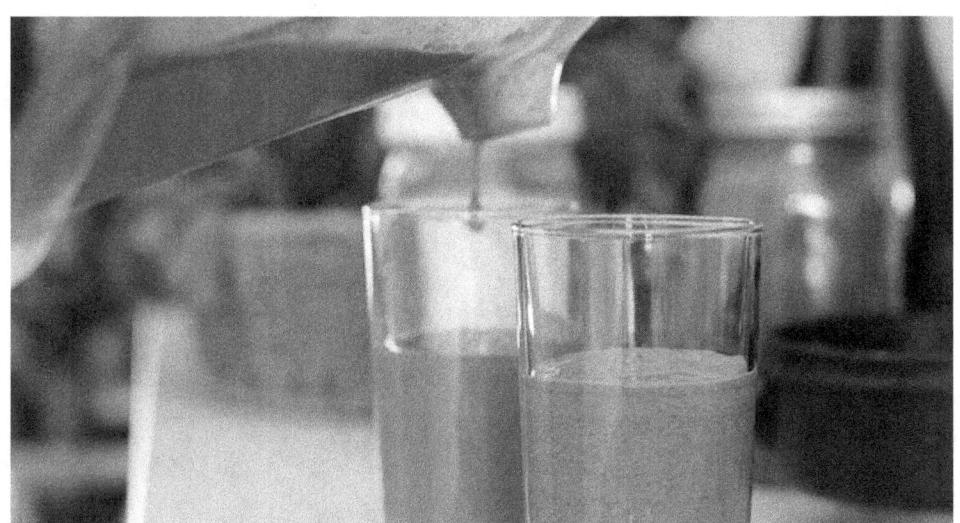

Ingredients:
- 10-15 cubes of ice (blend 1st and then add all other ingredients)
- 1 cup hemp milk
- 2 tbsp. almond butter
- 2 tbsp. pea protein or raw protein of choice
- 1 tsp. vanilla extract
- 1 tbsp. cacao powder or carob powder
- 2 tbsp. Dandy blend
- 1 tbsp. raw cacao nibs
- 2-3 dates or agave, stevia

Instructions:
1. Blend & serve!

Golden Spice Latte

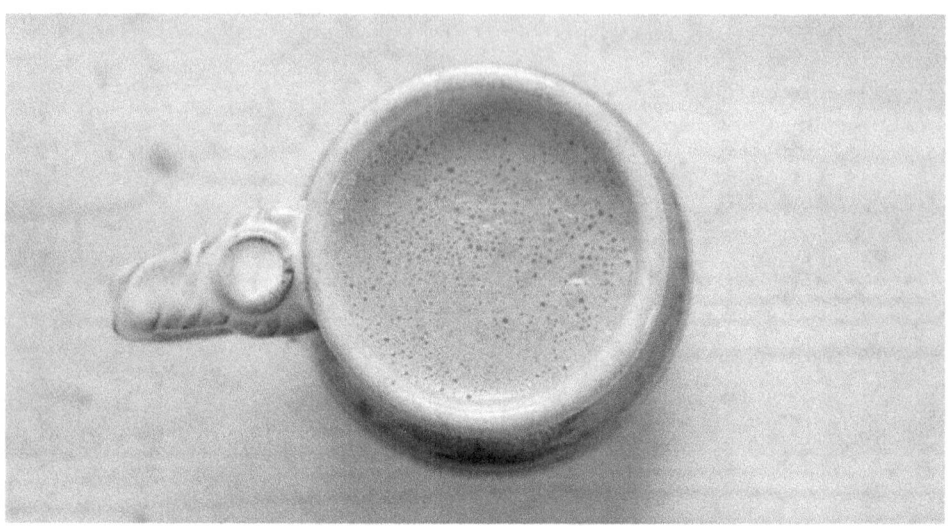

Ingredients:
- 1½ cups raw unsweetened almond milk, or raw nondairy milk of choice
- 1 Tbsp. coconut butter, softened
- 1½ tsp. Agave
- 1½ tsp. turmeric powder
- 1 tsp. Cinnamon
- ½ tsp. vanilla extract
- ¼ tsp. ginger powder

Instructions:
1. Place everything in your blender and blend to incorporate.

2. Transfer to your favorite mug and sip slowly.

Homemade Raw Coconut Yogurt

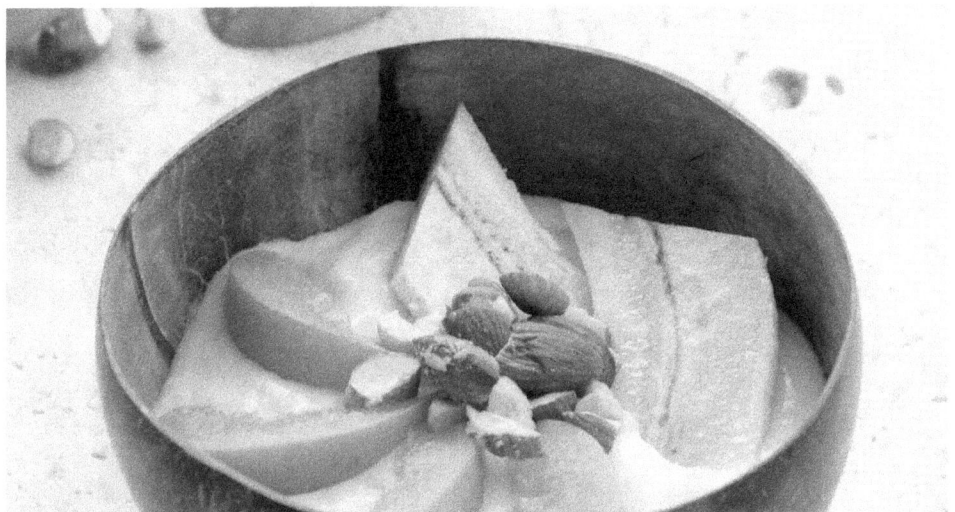

Instructions:
1. Open up four young coconuts and scoop out the flesh.

2. Pop the flesh in a sieve and rinse well, taking care to peel off any of the husk still attached.

3. Add the meat to a blender and empty in the contents of one dairy free probiotic capsule.

4. Whizz till nice and smooth.

5. Transfer the mixture into a jar or bowl, and cover the mouth loosely with a breathable fabric. Put the jar somewhere where it is reasonably warm, but not in direct sunlight.

6. Leave the mixture to culture for up to 12 hours, after this point, you can taste it to see if its ready, it should be a little sour.

7. Move to the fridge to stop the culturing process – you now have a perfectly natural, dairy free, probiotic filled yoghurt!

Overnight Breakfast Jars

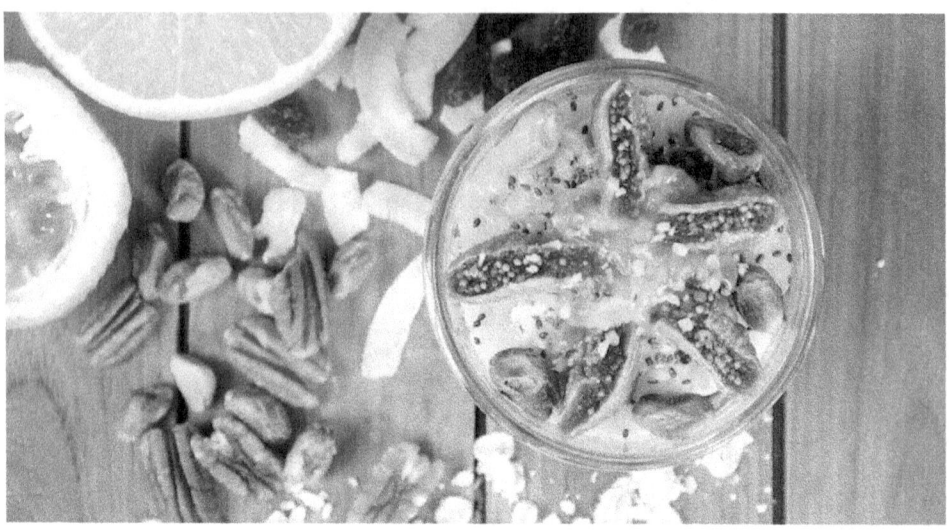

Ingredients:
- Raw oats
- Shredded coconut
- Raisins
- Flax seeds
- Banana sliced
- Pistachios
- Dried fig sliced
- Passion fruit
- Hemp seeds

Instructions:
1. Find a glass jar that you can use to fill- a small to medium size.

2. Simply top with raw almond milk once you are done with the layers and leave in the fridge overnight to set and soak.

3. In the morning the jar is ready to go! You can eat it straight as is or tip it upside down into a bowl and top with your favorite fruit.

Papaya Chia Pudding

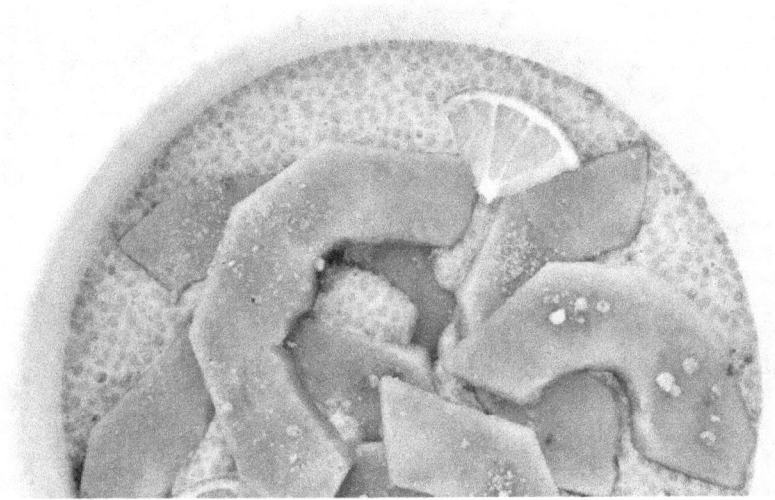

Ingredients:
- 2 cups unsweetened almond milk
- 6 tablespoons chia seeds
- Agave, to taste
- 1 small papaya, peeled and sliced
- Squeeze of lemon

Instructions:
1. Combine the almond milk, chia seeds, and agave in a glass container. Stir well until the chia seeds are mixed in. Stick in the fridge and let sit for a few hours or overnight. The chia seeds will expand as they continue to soak.

2. In the morning, give the pudding a good stir.

3. Drizzle the sliced papaya with a squeeze of lime and some more of the Agave Serve the pudding in bowls topped with the papaya, Enjoy!

Pumpkin Pie Persimmon

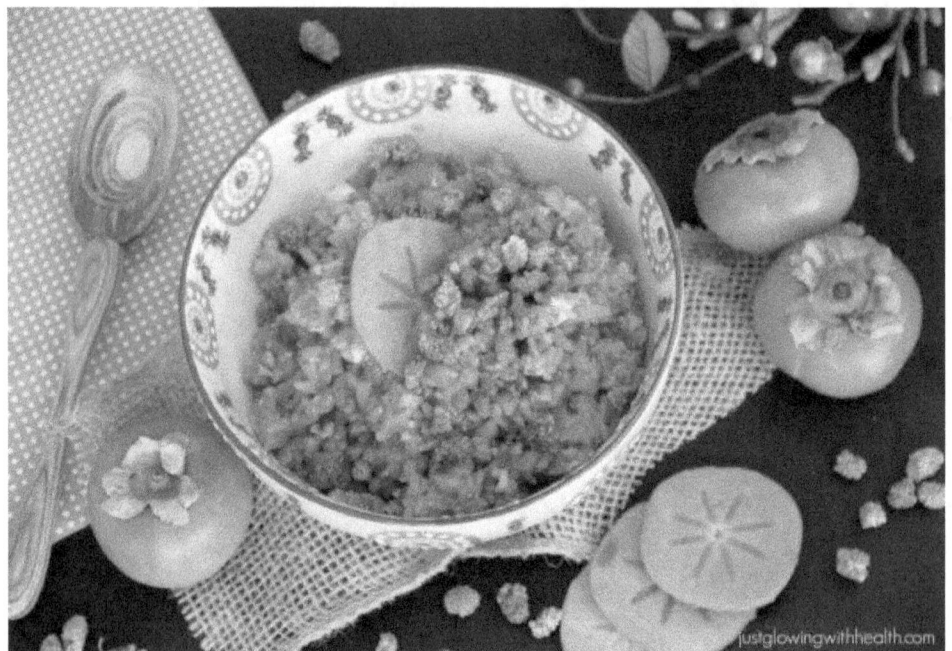

Ingredients:
- 5 Fuyu persimmons, chopped (tops removed)
- 1/3 cup pecans, soaked 6+ hours in filtered water then drained, rinsed and pat dry
- Handful dried mulberries
- 1/2 teaspoon pumpkin pie spice
- 1/8 teaspoon turmeric
- 5 dried apple rings
- Pinch of coconut sugar

Instructions:
1. Pulse all ingredients besides sugar in a food processor until it becomes a coarse mix. Scoop out into a bowl and top with more dried mulberries. Sprinkle coconut sugar on top.

Breakfast Muesli

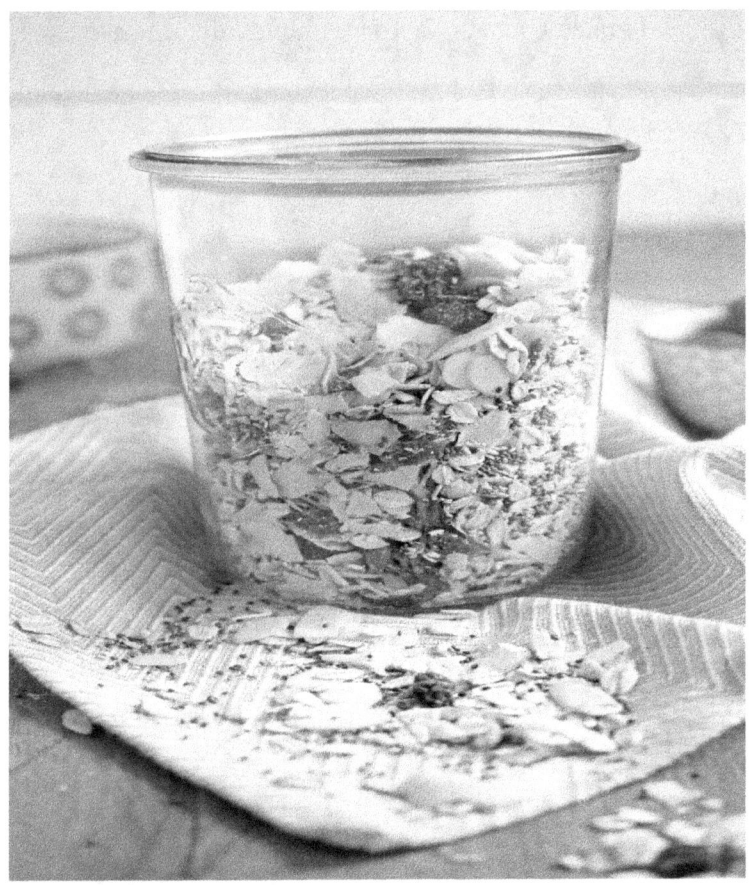

Ingredients:
- 3/4 cup nuts (raw)
- 10 dates (approximately, soaked and pitted)
- Optional: 2 tablespoons coconut oil
- 1 cup fresh fruit (mango, berries or banana works well)
- Optional: 1 tablespoon fresh raw grated coconut
- Splash nut milk (raw, to taste)

Steps to Make It Using a food processor, process the nuts and dates and coconut oil together until nuts are almost finely ground. 1. Combine in a bowl with fresh fruit and grated coconut. 2. Top with nut milk, to taste.

Raw Cinnamon Sugary Oatmeal

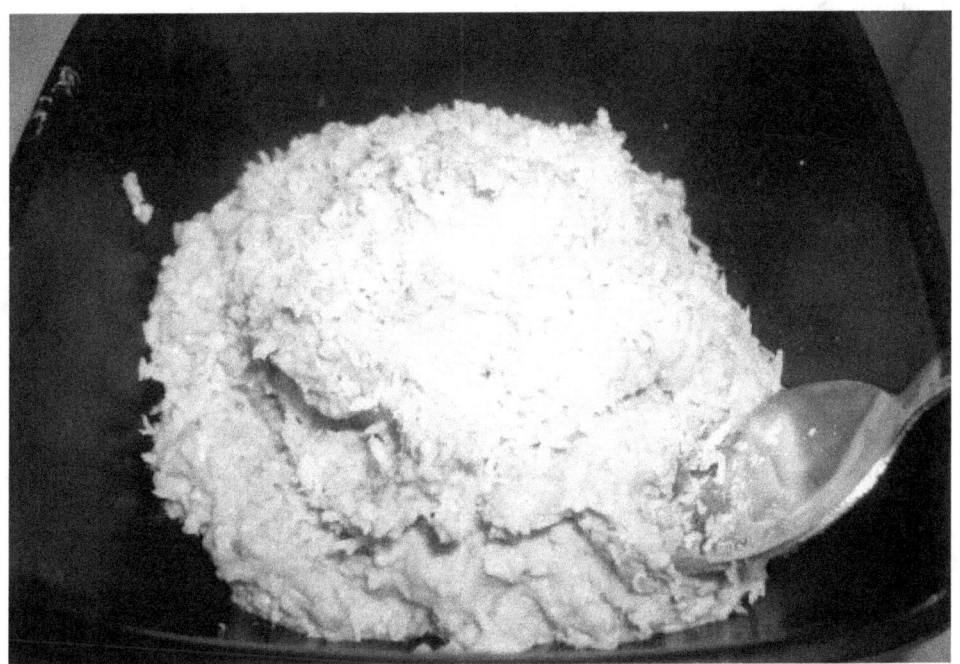

Preparation Time: 5 minutes
Servings: 1 to 2

Ingredients:
1 cup oat groats, soaked at least 12 hours 2 to 4 large medjool dates, pitted 1 teaspoon ground cinnamon Pinch salt 1/4 cup raw nondairy milk Stevia powder (optional) Dried coconut chips (optional)

Directions:
1) Rinse soaked oat groats well and transfer to a blender or food processor. Add the dates, cinnamon, salt, and raw nondairy milk. Blend on highest setting until the mixture turns very creamy.

Put in a bowl and enjoy! If you want it a little sweeter, add more dates or a heavy pinch of stevia at the end. For some extra flavor and crunch, add some coconut chips. If you like your oatmeal creamier, double or triple the amount of liquid used.

Coconut Chia Pudding

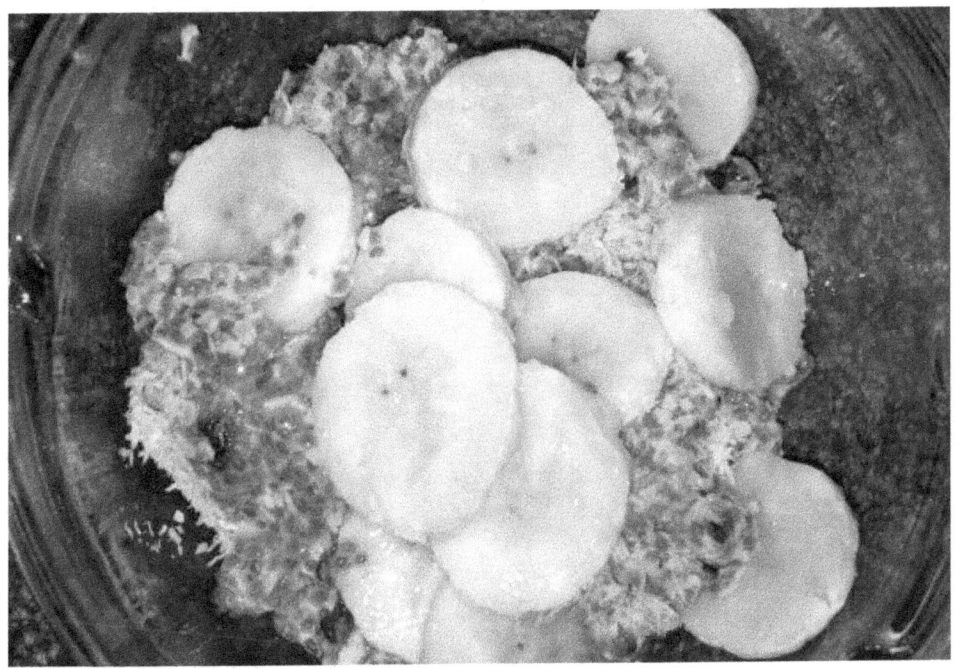

Preparation Time: 10 minutes
Servings: 2

Ingredients:
1/4 cup chia seeds
1/8 cup hemp seeds
1/4 cup raisins
3/4 cup nondairy milk (I use raw almond)
1/4 cup shredded coconut
1/8 cup cacao nibs 1 banana, sliced (or other fruit)
1-2 teaspoons agave, optional

Directions:
1. Combine chia seeds, hemp seeds, raisins, and milk in a bowl, and stir well to combine. Leave to sit for about 5 minutes to let the milk get absorbed. 2.

Gradually fold in the coconut and cacao. Top with fresh fruit slices, drizzle with agave, and enjoy!

Raw Banana Cocoflax Wrap

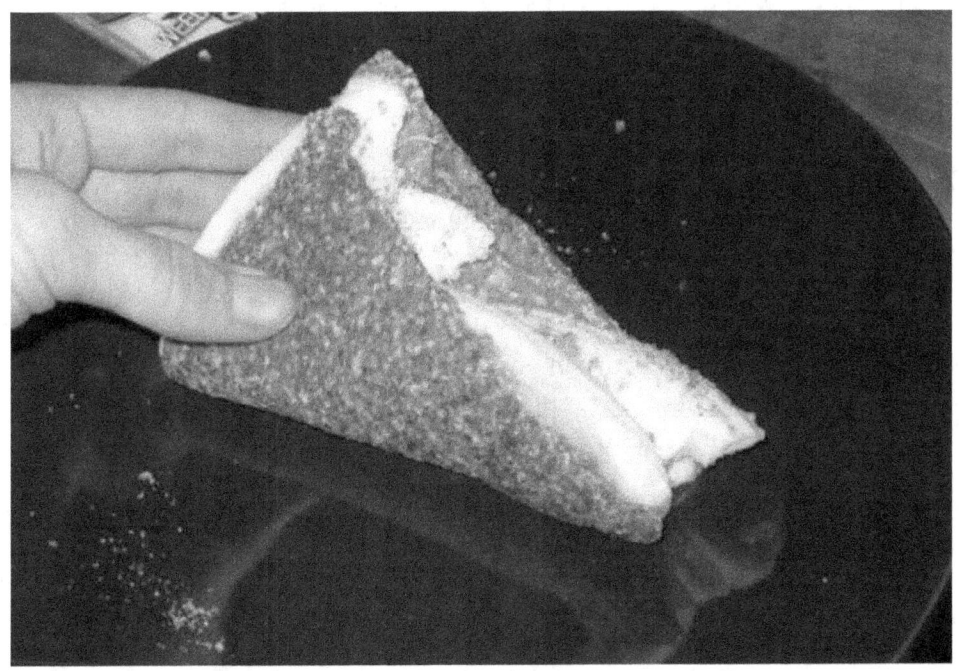

Preparation Time: 15 minutes
Servings: 4
"Cooking" Time: 4-6 hours

Ingredients:
1 cup coconut meat (about 1/2 coconut)
1/2 cup coconut water (not milk) I use plain water too a lot
1/4 cup ground flax (if you only have whole, grind it in a coffee grinder) a pinch or two of salt (important)
1 tablespoon almond butter (I used peanut butter in transition)
1 banana

Directions:
I eat this almost every morning, the other times I eat flax pancakes (recipe to come). Ok, the last two ingredients you use at the very end. So you can make the wrappers and while they are drying, you can go buy the other two

if you don't have em. Blend together (I use a food processor) the coconut meat, coconut water (or plain water), ground flax and salt. It should make a paste, not too wet, not to dry. Spread this on your non-stick dehydrator sheet. (I have fruit roll up sheets for my dehydrator and they work great.)

Make sure to spread this evenly, especially around the inside (I use a round dehydrator, so the "inside" is where the small vent hole is. You don't ave to worry about this with the square dehydrators.) Set you temp at 115 for an hour or two, then lower it to 105. After they are dry to the touch, flip them carefully. They will be moist underneath and you may tear one, but it's easy to fix (just spread it like glue to cover the tear). It takes practice. Then dehydrate until completely dry, if you want them crisp (they keep longer and in a zip lock on the counter). Or until dry, but still moist enough to be flexible (they keep in a zip lock in the fridge for just a few days this way).

Now! Spread your peanut butter and slice your banana on top. I usually sprinkle a little agave and extra flax on top.

Raw Granola

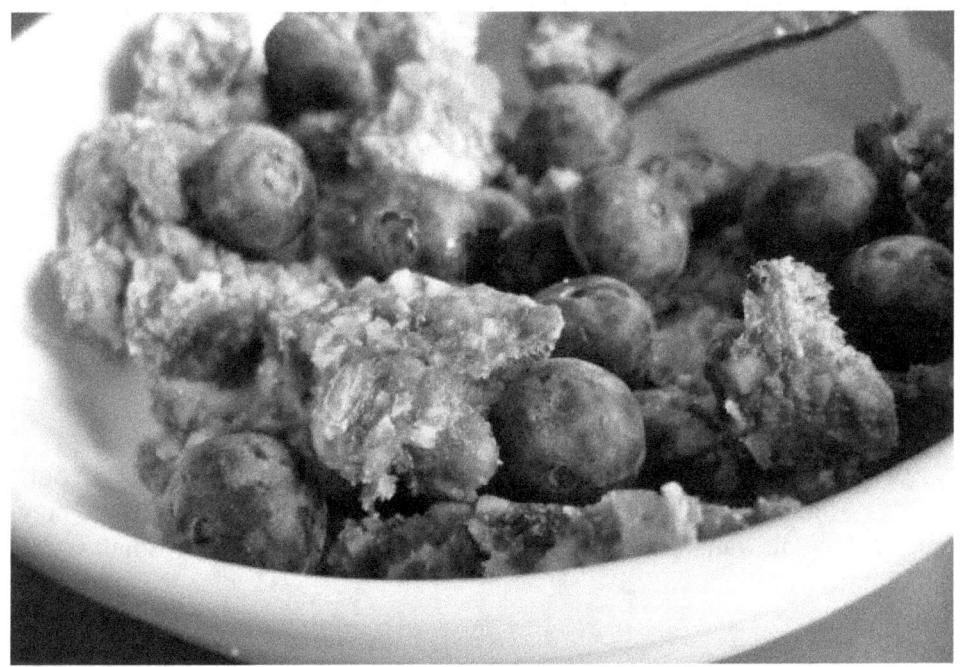

Preparation Time: 15 minutes
"Cooking" time: 12 hours
Servings: 4

Ingredients:
3 tablespoons water
1 tablespoon chia seeds
1-1/2 cups soaked almonds (soak at least 8 hours, then measure 1-1/2 cups)
1 cup soaked raw pecans
divided (soak at least 4 hours, then measure 1 cup)
2 tablespoons ground flaxseeds
1 teaspoon cinnamon
1/2 teaspoon sea salt
1 apple, peeled and chopped
1/4 cup agave syrup, nuts and/or dried fruit of your choice, to taste (optional)

Directions:
1. In a small bowl, mix together the water and chia seeds; set aside.

2. Finely chop soaked almonds (you could also pulse them in a food processor). You want to make sure they are finely chopped but not into a puree. Transfer almonds to a large bowl.

3. Finely chop 1/2 cup of the pecans and add to almonds. Add in ground flax, cinnamon, and salt; set aside.

4. In a blender or food processor, puree the apple, agave syrup, chia and remaining 1/2 cup soaked pecans. Add to the almond mixture. Stir in nuts and fruit.

5. Spread onto a dehydrator sheet and dehydrate overnight. (We did ours for 17 hours, but you can just see how dry it is the next morning and decide how much more you want to dry it for). Flip over and break into pieces half way through dehydration. Eat!

Raw Oatmeal with Cranberries

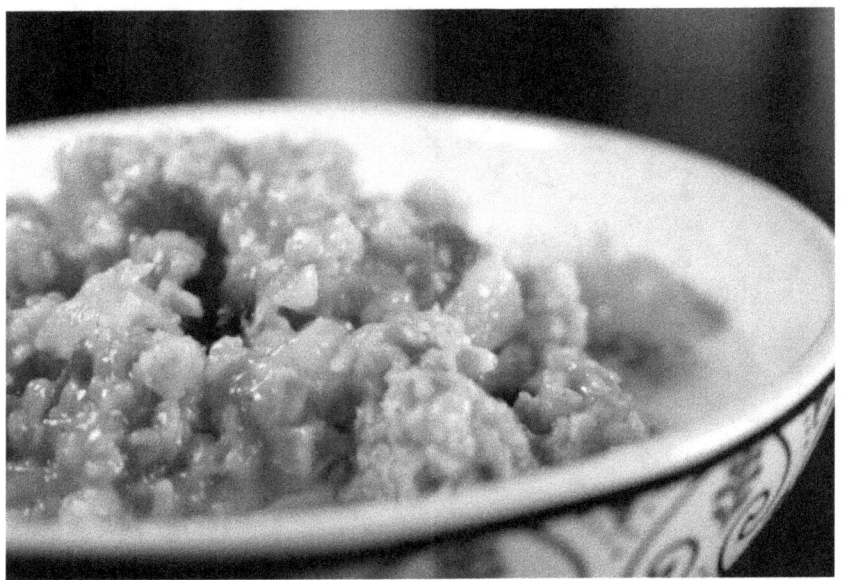

Preparation Time: 10 minutes
Servings: 1

Ingredients:
2 tablespoons cranberries
Apple juice
1 handful oat sprouts
1 handful wheat sprouts
1 banana

Directions:
1) Put about two tablespoons of cranberries in some apple juice to soak.

2) Take a handful of oat sprouts and a few handfuls of wheat sprouts and mix them together in a bowl. Peel the banana and mash in the bowl with the sprouts. Mix until you have a crunchy sprout banana consistency. You may have to add more sprouts. Strain the cranberries and stir in. Enjoy.

Raw Onion-Dill Bagels

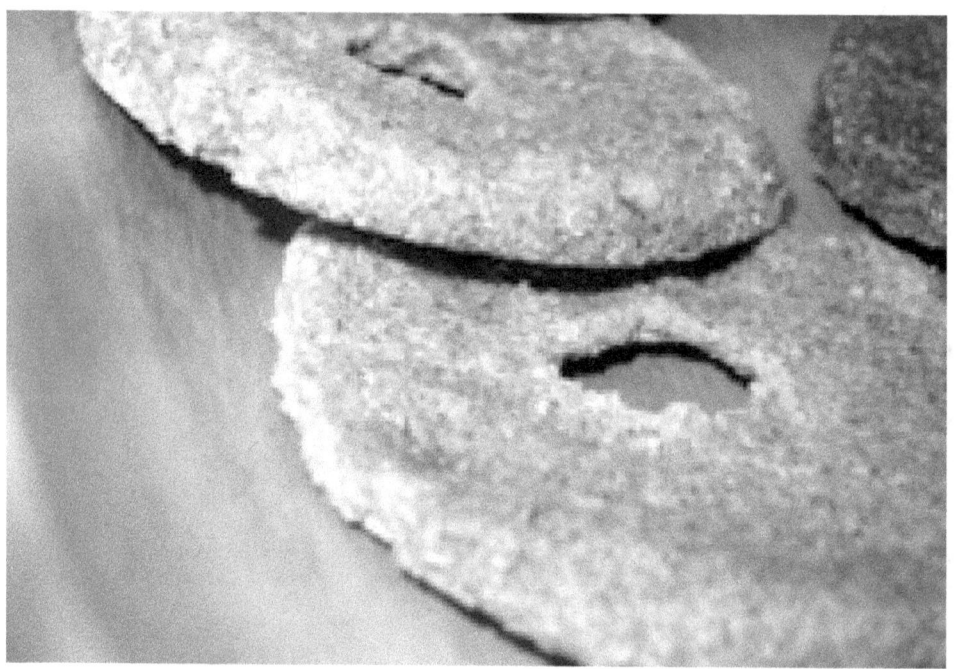

Preparation Time: 15 to 20 minutes
"Cooking" time: overnight (6 hours)
Servings: 4

Ingredients:
2/3 cup raw hulled sunflower seeds (I didn't soak)
1/3 cup raw golden flax seeds
1/3 cup chopped onion
1/3 cup fresh dill (or 3 tablespoons dried dill)
1/3 cup spelt berry rejuvelac
Pinch sea salt

Directions:
1) In a food processor, combine the sunflower seeds and golden flax seeds. Grind until a powder forms. Stir in the onion and dill and pulse until even.

Stir in the rejuvelac and sea salt and pulse a few more times until a dough forms.

2) Roll the dough into golf-sized balls. Flatten and place onto dehydrator sheets or parchment paper. If you want the hole in the middle, use a bottle cap to cut out the center, and pressing inward, close the gap to a smaller hole around the wide circle.

3) Dehydrate overnight (approx. 6 hours, give or take depending on your appliance), and enjoy fresh warm crisp on the outside, soft on the inside bagels for breakfast!

Raw Pancakes

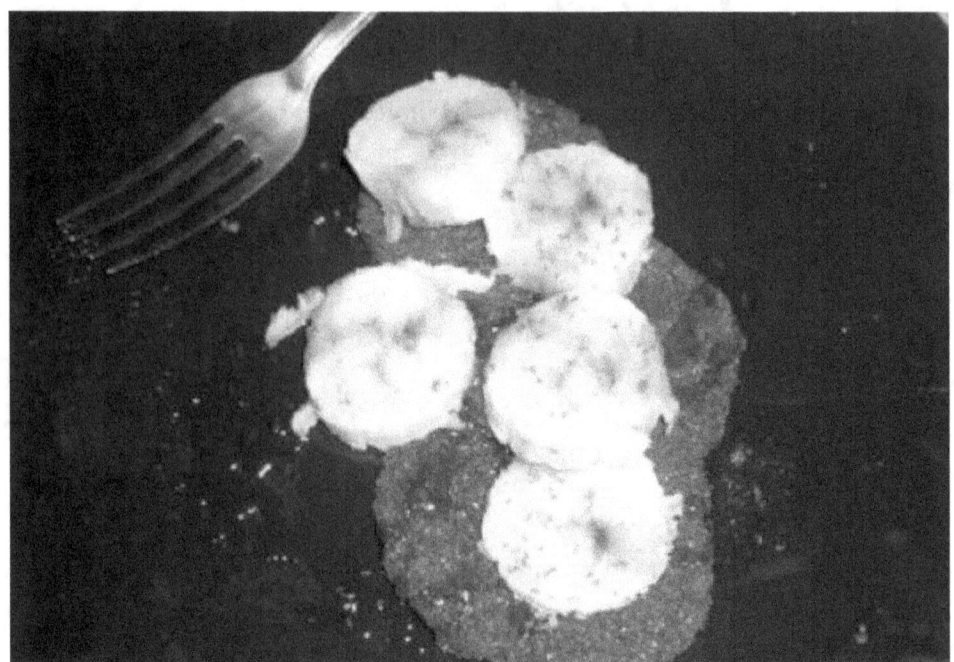

Preparation Time: 10 minutes
"Cooking" time: 10-15 minutes
Servings: 1

Ingredients:
1 cup ground flax
1 tablespoon coconut oil
1 banana or handful blueberries or carob chips
optional sprinkle salt
sprinkle cinnamon.

Directions:
1. Mix all ingredients in food processor.

2. Make little patties.

3. You can eat this now if you don't have a dehydrator, or set them in the sun. I only use a dehydrator because they get warm! Then you can add sliced fruit (I make mine plain flax and then add fruit on top) to the top. I mix agave with a tiny bit of vanilla. It is easy to over do the vanilla. But you could use orange extract or a fruit juice to mix and make flavored syrup too. This is so delicious! Enjoy!

Raisin Log

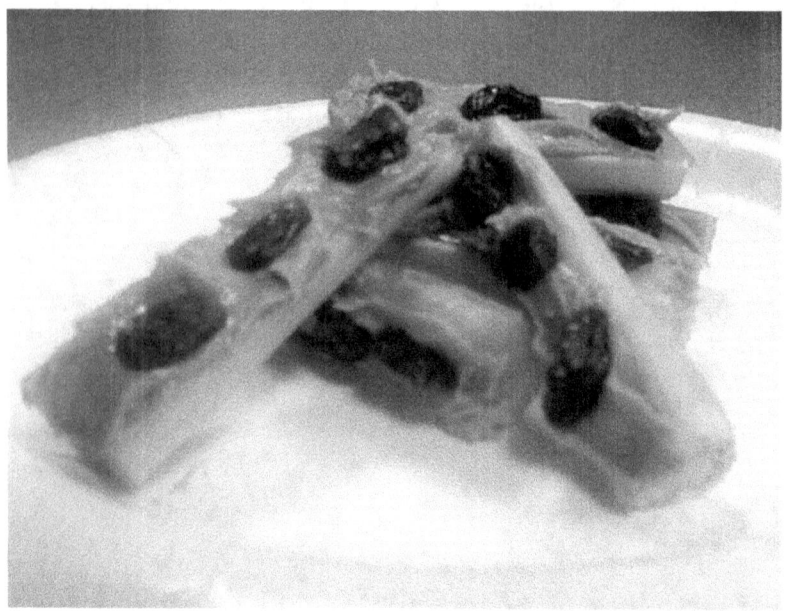

2 stalks celery
raw almond butter
raisins

Cut the celery in logs add almond butter top with raisins enjoy!

Strawberry Ravioli with Cacao Sauce: Valentine's Day Raw Food Breakfast

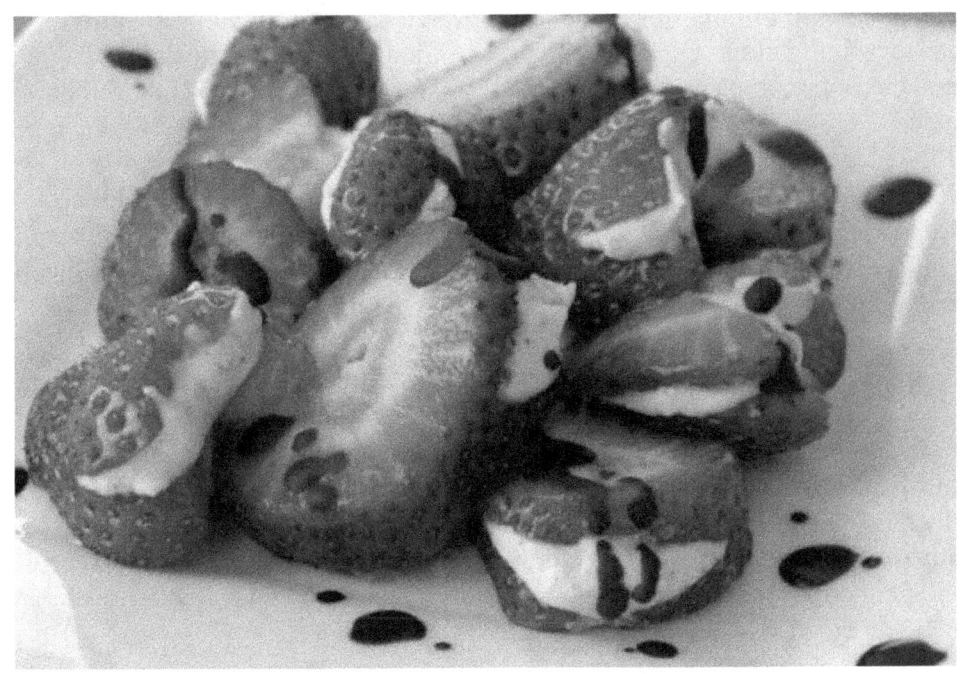

Preparation Time: 25 minutes
Servings: 1

Ingredients:
Pear Cream Filling:
1/2 cup cashews, soaked 2 to 4 hours (soaking recommended, but not necessary)
3/4 medium bosc or bartlet pear
1 teaspoon lemon juice
1 pint fresh strawberries

Cacao Sauce:
2 tablespoons shaved raw cacao butter
2 tablespoons raw cacao powder

1 teaspoon agave, or to taste

Directions:
1. Pear Cream Filling: In a blender—or Magic Bullet at my house—grind cashews into a flour. Coarsely chop pear. Add it and lemon juice to the cashew flour and blend until smooth. Set aside. (Pear Cream Filling can be made a day or two in advance.)

2. Strawberries: Cut 1/4" segments that can then be sliced to create a pocket. Depending on the size of your berries you may want to slice them lengthwise or crosswise, or alternate. To utilize the strawberry's natural heart shape remove the stem with a V cut and slice lengthwise.

3. Spoon filling into strawberry ravioli and place directly on a plate.

4. Cacao Sauce: In a double boiler—or your own version—melt the cacao over low heat (the cacao will melt without exceeding the critical 118 degrees). Add cacao powder and stir until dissolved. Add agave, keep stirring. (You may want to use more than a teaspoon of sweetener if you're a milk chocolate fan or your strawberries aren't sweet. Omit it if you prefer dark chocolate.)

5. Drizzle desired amount of cacao sauce over ravioli. Serve immediately, this is a great dish to share. Enjoy!

3.2 Lunch

Lettuce Wraps

Serves 4

Ingredients:
1/2 cup hemp seed
1/2 cup lemon juice
1/4 cup agave or a few drops of stevia (2-3)
1 1/2 tablespoon chopped ginger
1/2 tablespoon red chili
1 tablespoon Braggs Liquid Aminos
1 cup raw almond butter
1/2 head savoy cabbage, shredded
6 very large wild spinach leafs
1 carrot
1 ripe mango
1 handful cilantro leafs
1 handful torn basil leafs
Himalaya sea salt

Directions:

Cut the carrot into into matchstick-size pieces. Cut the Mango lengthwise into strips, about 1/4 inch (1 cm) thick.

In a Vita-Mix or high-speed blender, puree the agave (or stevia), lemon juice, ginger, red chili, and Braggs Liquids Aminos. Add the almond butter and blend at low speed to combine. You should get a rather thick consistency. (You may add water if it needs to be thinner)

In a bowl, mix the almond butter dressing with the cabbage. The best and easiest way is to do this with you hands or a large wooden spoon.

Now you need to roll the cabbage with dressing into a "lettuce" wrap. This is kind of tricky. Place the spinach leaf on a cutting board with the underside facing up. Then you put some of the cabbage mix on the leaf. Add some hemp seeds, a few sticks of carrot, a few pieces of mango, and a few leafs of cilantro and, basil.

Try to roll up and the spinach leaf, you might need to stick a cocktail stick in it to hold. Do this for all the other spinach leafs until the ingredients are gone.

Raw Food Balls

I love simple raw food recipes, this one especially. It is quick, easy, tasty and you can make it anywhere.

I came upon this recipe when I had to spend some time at a place without any blender or juicer with family that isn't eating a raw food diet. I didn't want to eat fruit only and I wanted to be very quick.

It's as simple as making coffee from powder (and it actually looks like it). You don't need any kitchen tools. I sometimes make this "smoothie" several times a day.

Ingredients:
1 large teaspoon of raw agave
2 teaspoons carob powder (or raw chocolate or mix)
1 teaspoon mesquite powder
2 teaspoons green powder (i.e. E3 Live Renew Me)
2 cups clean water
few drops liquids stevia

Directions:
Put the powders in a large glass. Add the agave. Fill the glass half way with water. Stir well until the agave is dissolved.
Add the rest of the water and stevia to taste.
That's it! This is a highly nutritious super foods smoothie.

Tips

1. I add the agave for taste. The stevia is for sweetness.

2. It looks like coffee. If your surrounded by cooked people, they'll assume you drink coffee.

3. If you don't have a glass and spoon available you can also put the ingredients in a water bottle and then shake.

4. To make other simple raw food recipes, you can add more super foods to this "smoothie" like cayenne, maca and raw chocolate.

5. You can pre-mix the ingredients and add them in a dispenser for baby formula powder

6. If you have a simple blender, such as a hand blander, you can substitute the agave for a banana and add hemp seed. They do require some short blending.

Fabulous Thai Coleslaw

Serves 4

Ingredients:

1/2 cup raw cashews
1/2 cup lemon juice
2 tablespoons chopped ginger
1/2 tablespoon red chili
1 1/2 tablespoon tamari
1 cup raw almond or peanut butter
1/2 head white cabbage, shredded
1/4 cup red cabbage, shredded
1/4 cup carrots, shredded
1 ripe mango, cut in small dices
1 handful cilantro leafs
1 handful torn basil leafs
Himalaya sea salt
2 tabelspoons agave nectar (or 1 tbsp and few drops stevia)

Directions

Cut the mango small cubes. Shred the cabbage and carrots.
In a Vita-Mix or high-speed blender, puree the agave, lemon juice, ginger, red chili and braggs aminos acid. Add the raw almond butter and blend at low speed to combine. To get a thick, cake batter-like consistency. Add water to thin if necessary.
In a bowl mix the cabbage and the raw almond butter mixture really well.
Add the raw cashews and mango pieces. Top with leafs of cilantro and basil and a few pieces of mango and or carrots for color.

Raw zucchini bread recipe

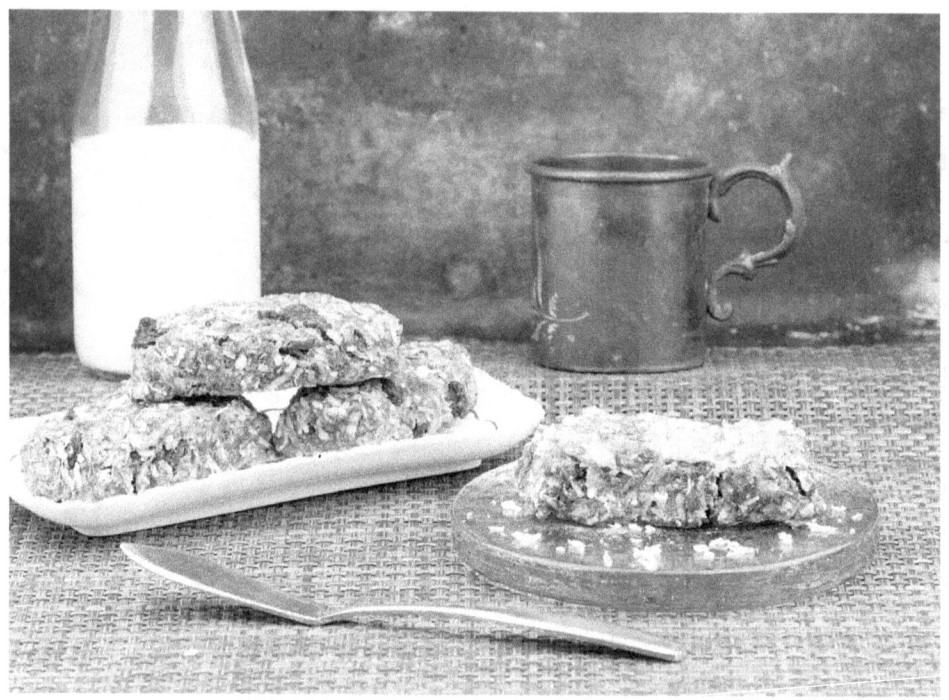

Ingredients:
3 cups grated zucchini
2 cups walnuts
1 1/2 cups dates
1/2 cup raisins
2 teaspoons cinnamon
1 teaspoon pure vanilla extract
1/2 teaspoon celtic sea salt
1/2 cup psyllium husk
1 cup shredded unsweetened coconut

Preparation Time 10 min
Wait Time 5 hours
Total Time 5 hours 10 min

Serving Size 10 servings
Shelf Life 5 days in fridge
Equipment Food Processor, Dehydrator

Directions:
1. Grate zucchini either by hand or in a food processor with a grating attachment. (Peeling is optional depending on how tough the peel is.) Place into a huge bowl and set aside.

2. Process walnuts in an empty food processor. Process into a fine meal.
3. Add dates, cinnamon and vanilla to nuts in food processor and process again until well mixed.

4. Remove mixture from food processor and add it to the big bowl that contains the zucchini. Combine with spoon or hands. (Mixture will appear dry but will moisture as you mix. Do not add any liquids.)

5. Stir in by hand raisins, coconut and psyllium husk.

6. Form into 10-11 loaves (see picture). Place on parchment paper. 7. Dehydrate on high for one hour. Reduce to 110 degrees for another five hours or until desired consistency is reached. 8. Store in refrigerator.

RAW CREAM OF MUSHROOM SOUP

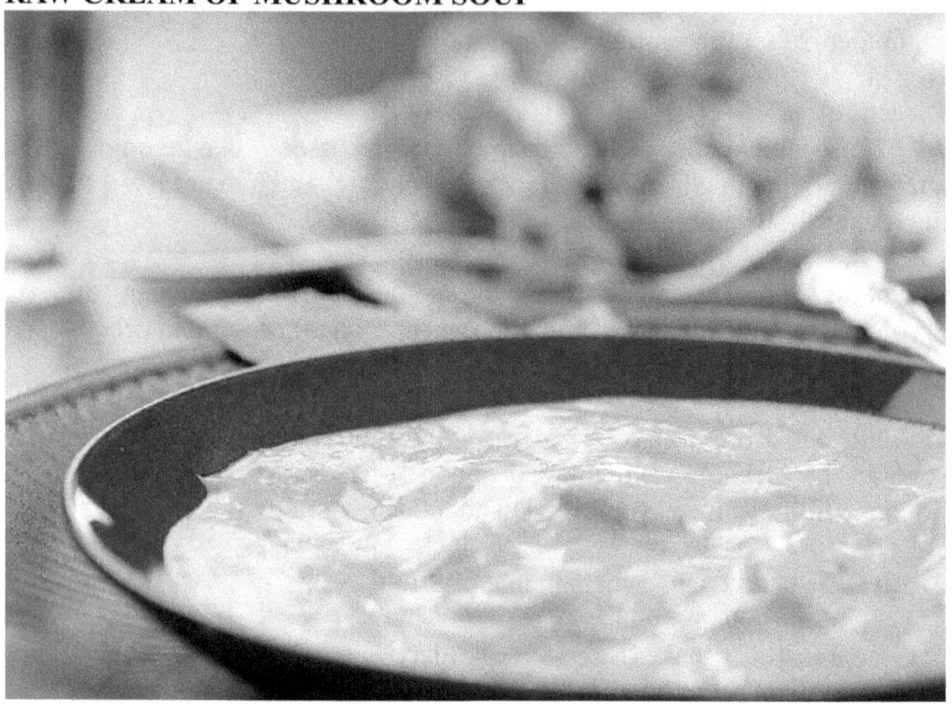

Ingredients:
1 1/4 cup chopped fresh mushrooms
1/3 cup cashews
1/4 to 3/4 cup water
1/4 teaspoon celtic sea salt
1/3 cup finely chopped fresh mushrooms (reserve - do not add to blender)
(and never use canned mushrooms for this part!!)

Preparation Time 5 min
Total Time 5 min
Serving Size 1 serving
Shelf Life Eat immediately

Equipment Blender
Directions:

1. Wash and dry your mushrooms. Chop 'em up a bit. (If you're using canned mushrooms, make sure to rinse and drain them. Pat dry with a clean tea towel.)

2. Add all ingredients (except the second amount of reserved finely chopped mushrooms) into your high-speed blender. Blend on high until very smooth and well-blended. Blend for an abnormally long time because you want this raw cream of mushroom recipe to be slightly warm when coming out of the blender.

3. Pour liquidy mushroom soup mixture into a bowl(s). Add remaining mushrooms and stir with a spoon. See what we're doing here? We're making a liquidy mixture and then adding some chunks to it to give it some texture and variety. That's the trick to all my raw soups.

4. Eat this raw cream of mushroom soup recipe immediately, while still warm from the blender!

RAW VEGAN TUNA AND MAYO COMBO

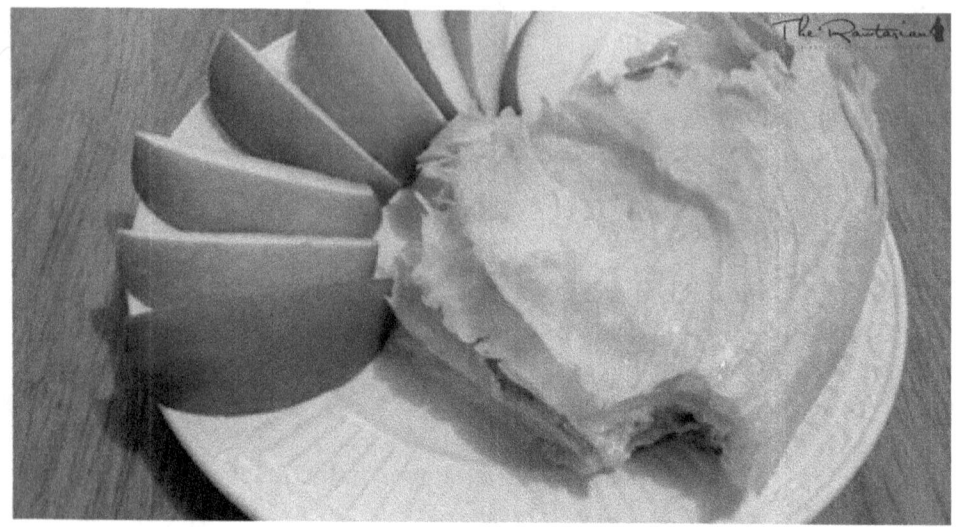

Ingredients:
1/2 cup walnuts
1/2 cup cashews
1 tablespoon lemon juice
1 tablespoon Braggs Liquid Aminos (or raw soy sauce or nama shoya)
1 tablespoon nutritional yeast
1 teaspoon coconut oil
1/2 a medium tomato
1/3 cup chopped carrot
1 tablespoon chopped white onion
1/8 teaspoon sea salt

Preparation Time 5 min
Wait Time 30 min
Total Time 35 min
Serving Size 4 servings
Shelf Life 4 days in fridge
Equipment Food Processor

Directions:

1. Throw walnuts and cashews into bowl. Cover with lukewarm water. Let soak for at least 1/2 hour. Discard water. Rinse well. Drain. You should now have some slightly wet nuts. Pat them dry with a clean tea towel. The purpose of soaking/rinsing is to soften the nuts and remove the enzyme inhibitors, which have a bitter taste. This recipe is a little more moist than some nut pates, so be sure not to be sloppy and add too much nut water.

2. Place all ingredients in your food processor. (Do not use your blender for this.)

3. Process until very well processed, like in the above photo. You will need to stop every so often and scrape the sides of your food processor. You'll know you're done when the consistency is like the above photo.

4. Once well blended, consume immediately. Store leftovers in the fridge.

RAW TACO MEAT RECIPE

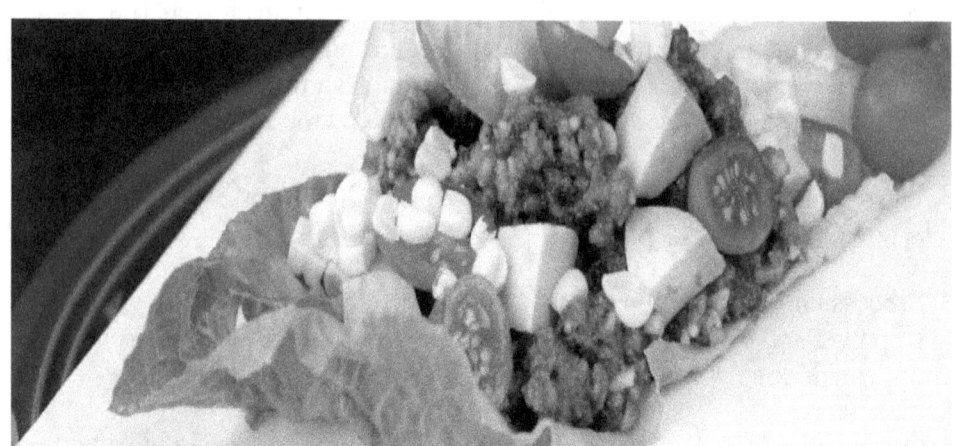

Ingredients:
1 cup walnuts
10 sundried tomatoes, soaked for at least one hour, preferably a few hours.
1-2 tablespoons olive oil
Chili powder (start with 1/4 tablespoon, then add more to taste)
Cayenne powder (start with 1/8 teaspoon or less!) (This measurement has been revised and is better now!)
1/2-1 tsp sea salt

Preparation Time 5 min
Total Time 5 min
Serving Size 3 servings
Shelf Life 4 days in fridge
Equipment Food Processor

Directions:
1. If you are using dry sundried tomatoes, soak your sundried tomatoes for at least one hour. Drain and pat dry before using. (If your sun-dried tomatoes are packed in oil you don't need to do this.)

2. Simply add all ingredients to the food processor and blend until it become the consistency of the photo above.

Raw mayonnaise recipe

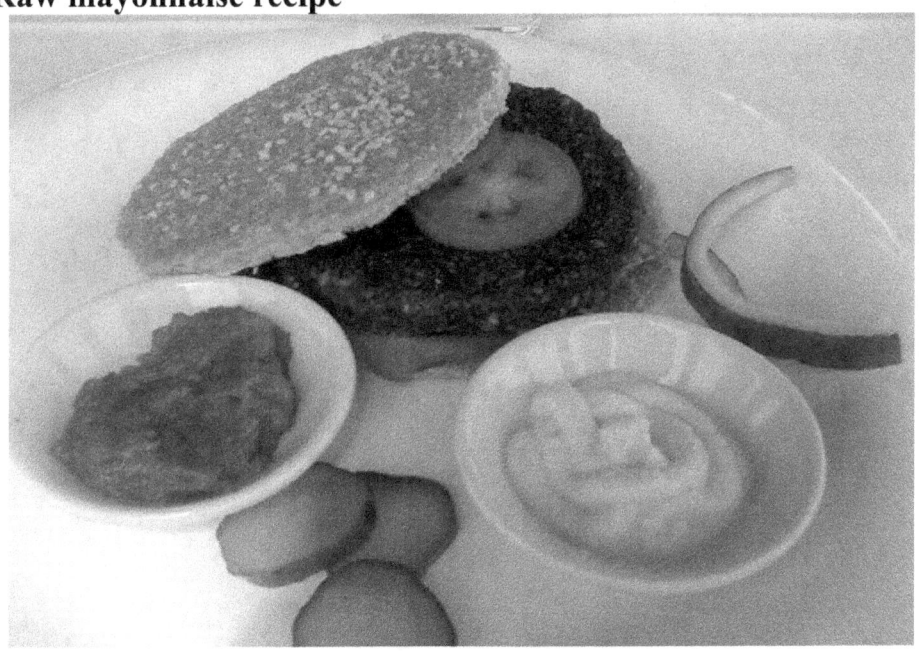

Ingredients:
3/4 cups water (or less)
1 1/2 cups of macadamia nuts (expensive but worth it)
3 tablespoons olive oil
2 tablespoons apple cider vinegar
1 teaspoon italian spices (basil, thyme, oregano or combo of all - whatever you have)
1/2 teaspoon sea salt dash of cayenne

Preparation Time 5 min
Total Time 5 min
Serving Size Varies
Shelf Life 4 days in fridge

Equipment Blender

Directions:
1. Throw everything in the blender and just BLEND until smooth!

Raw ketchup recipe

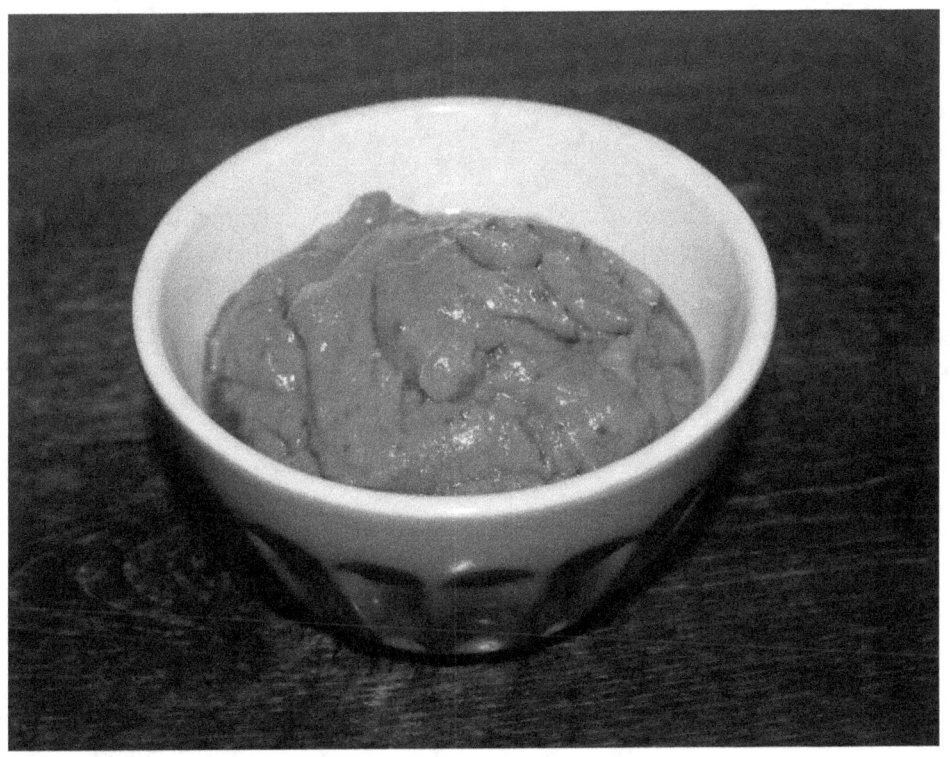

Ingredients:
1 1/2 cups of diced tomatoes
3 tablespoons dates (do not soak)
1/4 cup olive oil
1 teaspoon sea salt
1 tablespoon apple cider vinegar
1/2 cup sun dried tomatoes (dry - do not soak)

Preparation Time 5 min
Total Time 5 min
Serving Size Varies
Shelf Life 5 days in fridge

Equipment Blender

Directions:

1. Blend everything in the blender except the sun dried tomatoes. Add the sun dried tomatoes in last and blend until you get a ketchupy consistency.

2. Ketchup is complete!

3. Serve on veggie burgers and don't forget your raw mayonnaise (yummy)!! Or serve this raw ketchup recipe on top of raw macaroni and cheese. :)

Spicy Peanut Sauce

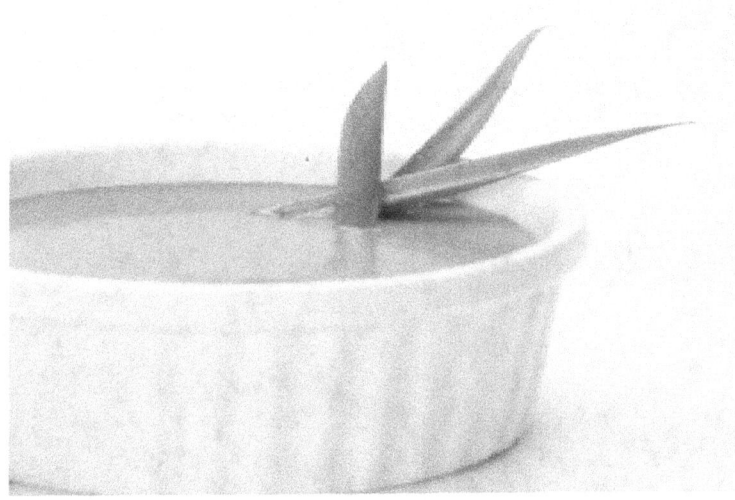

This is the PERFECT combination of sweet and spicy. Fabulous addition to spring rolls or cabbage wraps. Just dip and enjoy!

Equipment Needed Blender
Serves 6

Ingredients :
1/4 cup toasted sesame oil
1/2 cup peanut butter, organic, raw
2 Tbsp lemon juice, freshly squeezed
2 Tbsp agave nectar
1 Tbsp chipotle peppers, diced
1/2 cup water, filtered

Methods/steps:
1. Add water and all remaining ingredients into blender and blend. Add more or less water for desired consistency.

2. Store in air tight container for up to 5 days in refrigerator.

Raw sour cream recipe

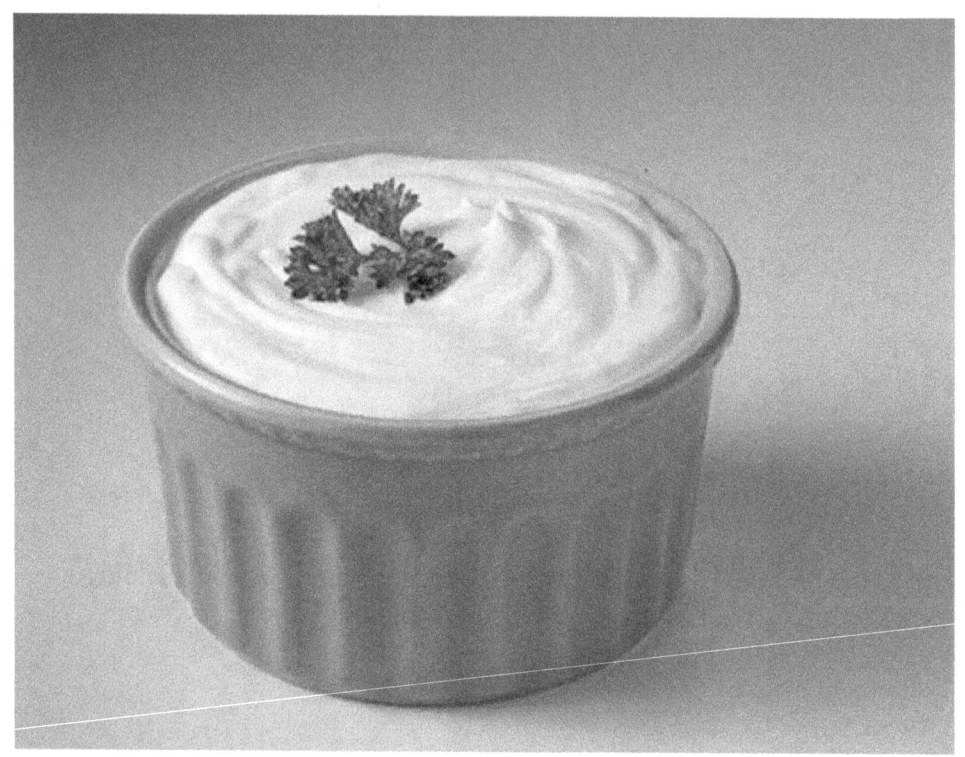

Ingredients:
1 cup of cashews (soaked and rinsed)
1/2 cup of water
1/4 cup of lemon juice
3/4 teaspoon onion powder
1/2 teaspoon celtic sea salt
Preparation Time 5 min
Total Time 5 min
Serving Size Varies
Shelf Life 4 days in fridge
Equipment Blender
Directions:

1. If you are wise and patient, soak your cashews first and then rinse them before blending. If you are impatient and have a high-speed blender, just throw dry cashews in your blender.

2. Add all ingredients, including cashews, into your blender.

3. Blend until smooth.

4. Transfer to a bowl and then chill in fridge for at least 2 hours.

5. Enjoy on raw vegan tacos or as a dip!

Sun-dried Tomato Spread and Dip

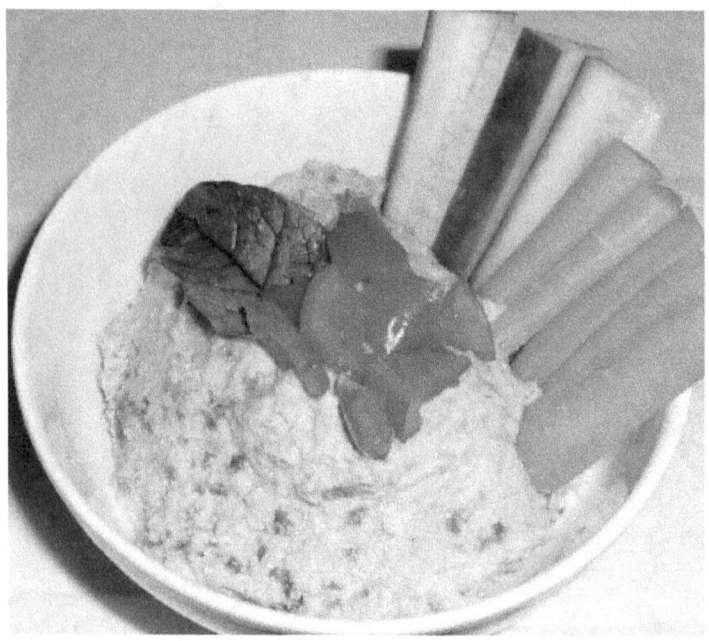

Meet my replacement for Ranch Dressing, Mayonnaise and Rice... yep you heard me! I make a batch of this every week and use it as a veg dip, sandwich spread and rice replacement.

This diverse concoction has a lot of flavor without the sundried tomatoes being too overpowering. But my favorite use for this is to replace sushi rice.

Equipment Needed Food Processor
2 Makes 1-2 c spread, or enough for 1 vegan sushi recipe

Ingredients:
3/4 c Cashews, soaked overnight
1/3 c Sundried Tomatoes, chopped
1 tbls Nutritional Yeast Flakes (optional)
1/2 of a Lemon juice * Pinch of Celtic Sea Salt
1/2 c Filtered Water
Methods/steps:

1) Add all the ingredients in a food processor and blend until a thick creamy consistency.

Raw Onion Bread Recipe

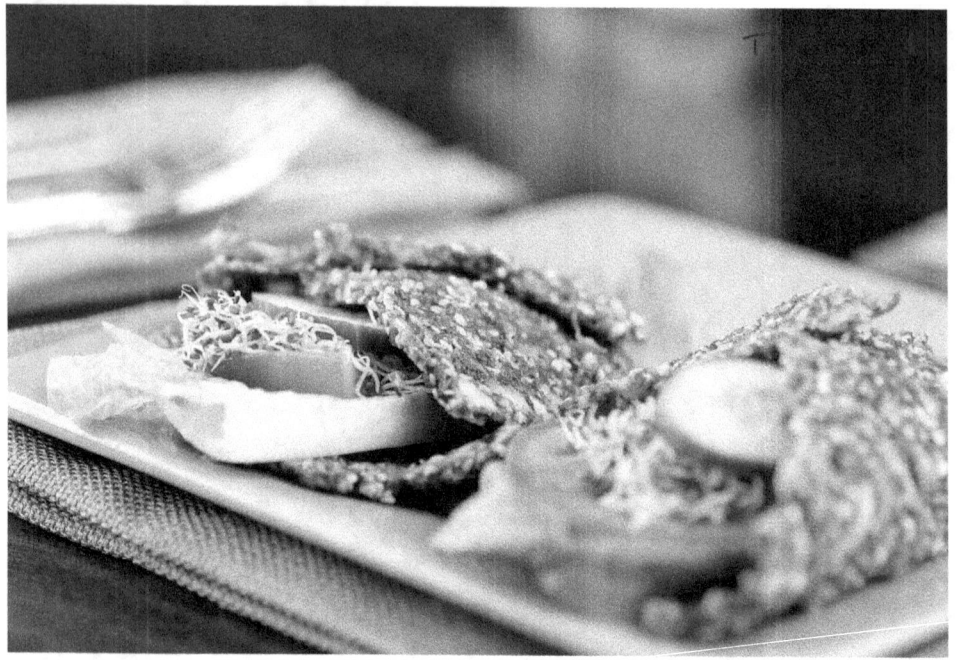

Ingredients:
3 massive, huge sweet white onions (2.5 pounds)
1 cup ground sunflower seeds (you can grind them yourself using a coffee grinder)
1 cup ground flax seeds (you can grind them yourself using a coffee grinder)
1/3 cup olive oil
3 1/2 tablespoons of Braggs Liquid Aminos, tamari or nama shoyu

Preparation Time 7 min
Wait Time 6 hours
Total Time 6 hours 7 min
Serving Size 6 wraps (3 trays)
Shelf Life 4 days in fridge
Equipment Food Processor   Dehydrator

Directions:

1. Peel onions, place in food processor and process in your food processor until small but not mushy. (Do not use a high-speed blender.):

2. Place onions in a large mixing bowl. Add everything else! Mix with a spoon. If it's dry and won't mix, you can add a small splash of water (ex. 1 tbsp), but I doubt you'll need to add any water at all.:

3. Spread onto dehydrator trays. Use parchment paper (not wax paper because it'll melt and stick!!!) or teflex sheets as a base. This raw onion bread recipe makes three Excalibur trays.:

4. Dehydrate for 1 hour at 120 degrees, then reduce to 105 degrees and dry for another 6 hours. Once the crackers start drying out and holding together, score them with a knife.:

5. At some point you'll want to flip them over, remove the parchment paper and finish dehydrating them, maybe for another 4 hours or so. I like them to be a bit chewy. Just try nibbling on this raw onion bread recipe and see whether you want it crispier. Dehydrating times can vary greatly, so trust YOUR judgment.

6. Enjoy this raw onion bread recipe!

3.3 Entrees

Symptoms of parasite infestations can be quite varied and mimic a large number of other disorders. Following is a partial list of possible symptoms:

Vegan Cheese Recipe

Here's an excellent vegan cheese recipe. It tastes just like young goat cheese. Perfect in salads, as a spread or dip. Made with pine nuts, garlic and fresh chives.

Ingredients:
1 cup pine nuts (soaked in water for 2 hours)
1 tbs extra virgin & cold pressed olive oil
1 tbs lemon juice (about juice of 1/2 large lemon)
1/2 tsp sea salt
1 glove garlic
pepper
fresh chives (optional)

Preparation:
Put all ingredients - except the chives - in your hand blender or food processor. Blend well, until smooth.

Take a few stalks of chives and cut them with a sharp knife or scissors into small pieces. Add to the cheese and blend in with fork.

Tip

This cheese recipe is great as a dip with carrots, spread on cucumbers or in your salad.
You can even make small balls with two spoons and roll them into herbs. Now you have cute little goat cheese balls (like little mozzarella cheeses) with herbs. These are fantastic in your salad.
You can keep the cheese in your fridge in a glass jar for 3 days.

Spaghetti al Marinara

Serves 4

Ingredients:

Spaghetti:
3 yellow summer squash or zucchini
Marinara Sauce:
6 large tomatoes
5 sun dried tomatoes
2 garlic cloves
1/2 bunch fresh basil
2 tablespoons oregano
1 tablespoon freshly ground black pepper
1/4 cup onion, chopped
1/2 cup cold-pressed olive oil
1/4 cup lemon juice
4 dates, pitted
1 teaspoon Himalayan sea salt

Directions:

For The Pasta:
There are several ways to make pasta from a squash. I use a julienne peeler (sold at better kitchen appliances stores). It looks like a cheese slicer or potato peeler. With this fancy but inexpensive and easy to use tool you make the most beautiful raw spaghetti strings in seconds.

You can also use an ordinary (potato) peeler: Peel thin slices of the squash, then with a fork or knife, create thin strands of "pasta".

Another way is using a kitchen tool often used in the raw food kitchen and by chefs: a spiralizer. Cut the zucchini in about four pieces and by putting them in the mandolin, you can create beautiful thin angel hair pasta. But I have to be honest, it never works for me...

Put the pasta strands in a bowl and sprinkle with a mixture of olive oil and some salt. Set aside.

For The Marinara Sauce:

Put all ingredients in a high speed blender and blend until creamy. Add purified water if you feel the consistency is too thick.

For serving:
Take off the excess oil of the pasta. Put the pasta on a plate and top with the sauce. You may add additional toppings such as slice olives, chopped tomatoes, onions or basil leafs.

Avocado Carrot Soup

Serves 2

Ingredients:

1 Avocado
2 Medium Carrots
1/4 cup Almond or Sesame Milk
1 teaspoon Ginger (finely chopped)
1/4 Lemon
2-4 drops Stevia or 1 tablespoon of coconut sugar, or agave (optional)
pinch cayenne pepper
Pure Water (until you get desired consistency)

Directions:

Put all ingredients in a high speed blender and mix well. Add some purified water or carrot juice if the consistency is too thick.

Gazpacho Soup
Serves 2

Ingredients:

for the soup:
4 tomatoes, diced
1/2 medium white onion, diced
1 glove garlic, peeled and minced
Lemon juice to taste
1 cucumber, peeled and chopped
for serving:
4 tablespoons freshly chopped cilantro
1 scallion (green part), finely chopped, for garnish
1 red bell pepper, seeded cored, and diced
1 table spoon raw virgin olive oil
1/4 cup mango, diced in small cubes

Directions:

Place all ingredients a blender and puree. Strain (vegetable press is easiest) to remove any vegetable pieces and pits that are not fully liquefied (like tomato skins or seeds). Alternatively, if you have a juicer, you can also put all ingredients in the juicer, using a coarse screen.

Chill overnight, if time permits. Before serving, sprinkle the chopped scallions, olive oil, some finely cut cilantro and mango.

Raw Olive Tapenade

Serves 6-8

Ingredients*:*
1 glove garlic
1 cup black olives (i.e. Natures First Law Italian)
Sea Salt & pepper
Olive Oil
Juice of 1/2 Lemon

Directions:

Take pits out of olives (if necessary). Place garlic, olives, olive oil and some juice in a blender and blend (I prefer not too fine). Add salt & pepper and lemon juice to taste and add some more olive oil to make the tapenade nice and smooth.

Raw Avocado Cream Zucchini Pasta

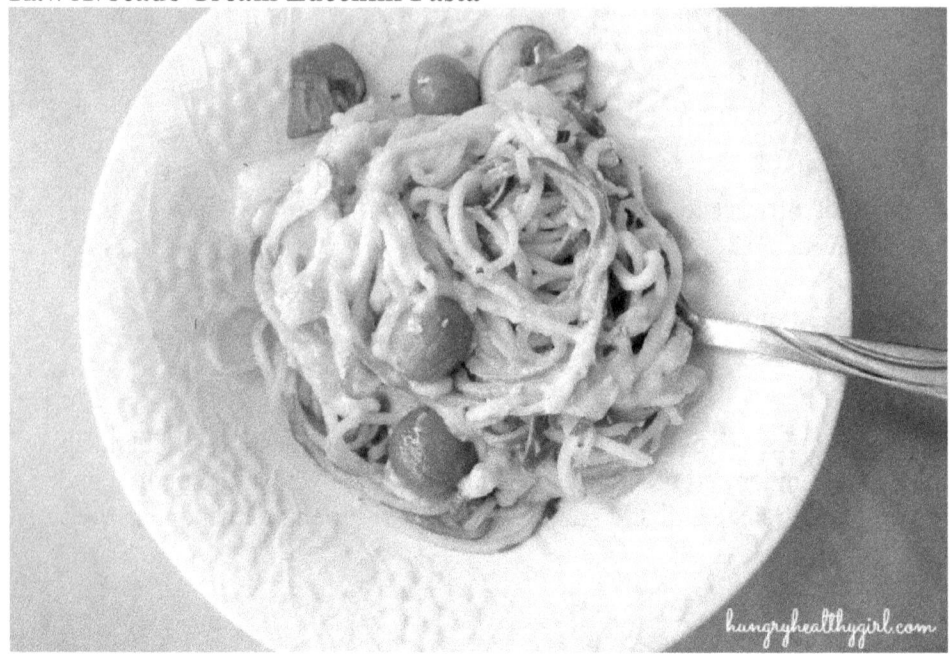

Preparation Time: 15
Servings: 2

Ingredients:
2 zucchini
1 carrot
1 small red bell pepper
1/2 cup snow peas
1/2 Hass avocado (or 1 smaller one)
1/4 cup water
1/2 lemon, juice and zest
1/4 teaspoon thyme
1/4 teaspoon rosemary
1/4 teaspoon sea salt
1/4 teaspoon black pepper

Directions:
1) Julienne the zucchini and carrot into a medium bowl. Chop pepper and snow peas and toss with the veggie "pasta".
2) Blend all the sauce ingredients in a food processor or blender until creamy.
3) Add the sauce to the pasta and toss to combine.
4) Serve on a bed of lettuce (optional).

Pasta will keep in the refrigerator for about 3 days, and the avocado will stay green.

Raw Burger

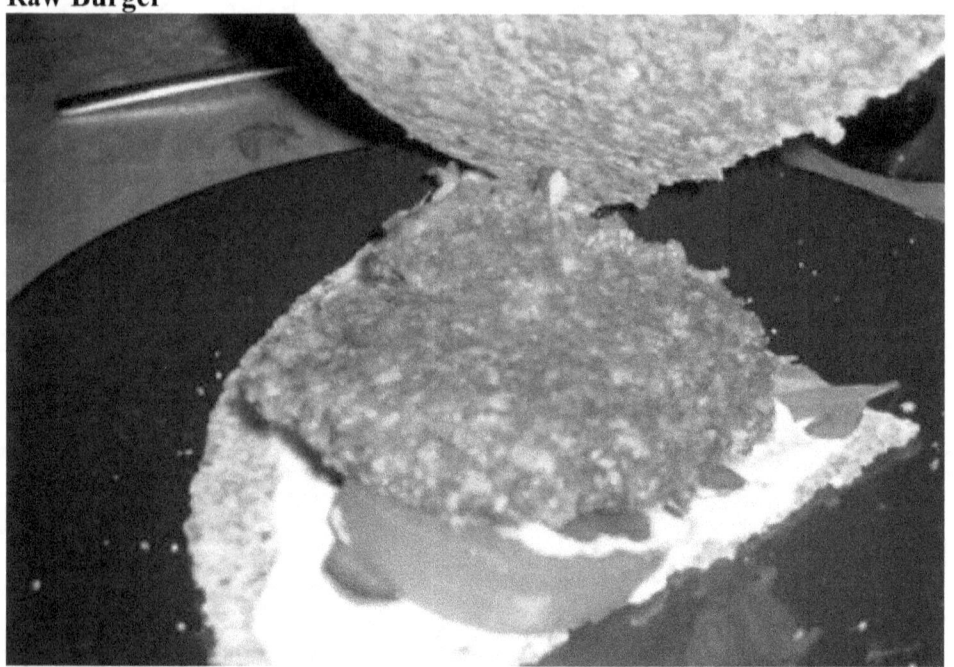

Preparation Time: 20 minutes,
Servings: 4 to 6
Prepping Time: 5 hours

Ingredients:
1/2 cup soaked sunflower seeds 4 carrots, shredded 1/2 onion 1/4 cup mushrooms 1/2 red pepper handful cauliflower or beets 1/2 jalapeno (omit if you don't want spicy burgers) Pinch salt Pinch EACH: cumin, paprika, coriander, sage, black pepper, turmeric

Directions:
1) Pulse all ingredients in a food processor until well mixed. Continue processing, adding a little water at a time until a not-too-wet dough forms. 2) Form patties and place on non-stick sheets or fruit roll up sheets. Dehydrate for 2 hours at 115 degrees Fahrenheit. The moisture content keeps the temp a

little lower than that inside the machine. 3) After two hours, reduce heat to 105 degrees Fahrenheit and continue drying 1 to 2 additional hours, until dry and firm enough to flip.

You can speed it up, by taking the flipped patties off of the non stick and placing them on the screen or mesh. Two more hours like this, or until you like. You can eat these immediately if you don't mind the soft mushy texture, but the dehydrator helps to form a solid patty. Be sure not over dry. Time varies per machine. You want them a little moist inside. Store in airtight container and eat in 3 to 4 days.

Cool, Creamy, Cauliflower Soup

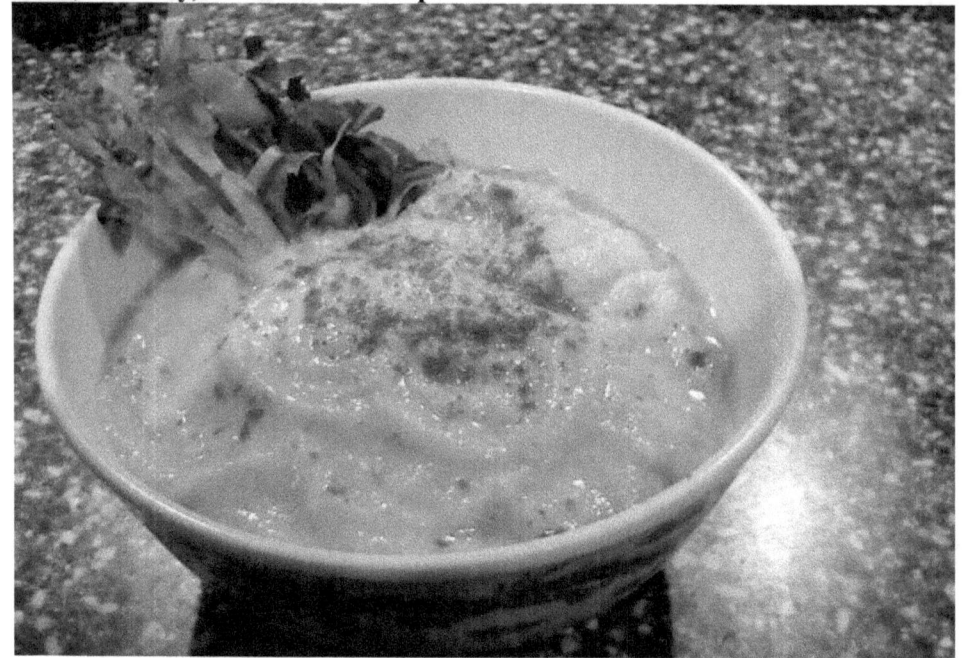

Preparation Time: 15 to 20 minutes
Servings: 2 Cooking Time:

Ingredients:
2 cups cauliflower, minced 1/2 avocado 1 cup raw nondairy milk (I use homemade almond) 1/2 cup coconut water 1/2 small onion 5 to 6 cherry tomatoes 1/2 cup red pepper, chopped 3 cloves garlic, minced Himalayan salt, to taste Curry powder, to taste Dill weed, to taste Cayenne pepper, to taste Ground black pepper, to taste Paprika, to taste.

Directions:
1) Put all ingredients in food processor. Blend until smooth. Garnish with a little paprika. Source of recipe: I have been trying to go more raw recently. I saw a recipe for a cauliflower soup and decided to make my own version. I didn't measure the spices so put in as much or as little as you would like.

RAW Creamy Mushroom Soup

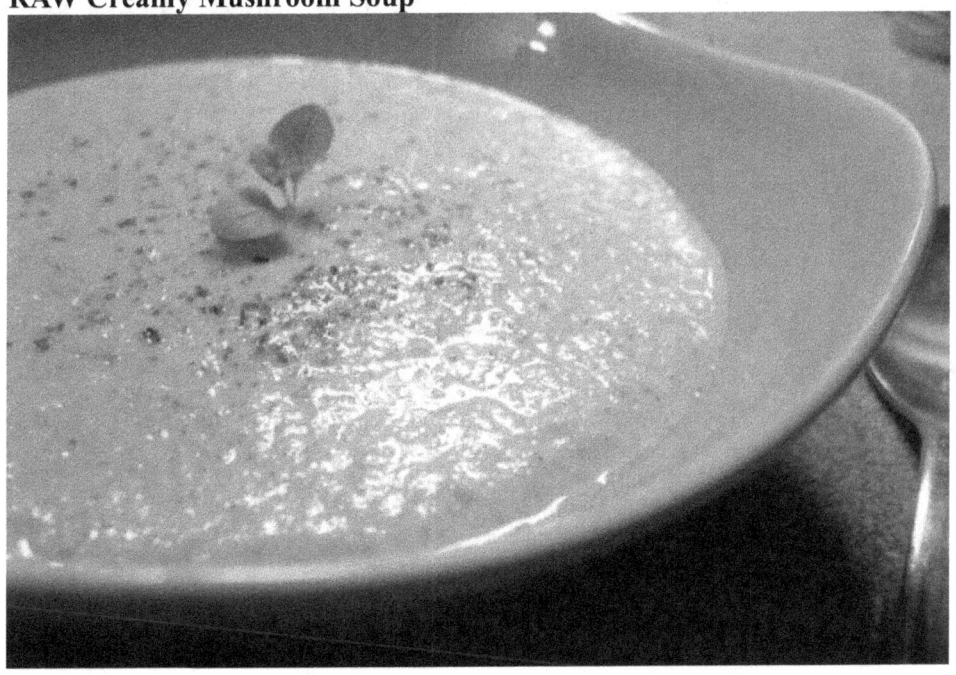

Preparation Time: 6 minutes
Servings: 2

Ingredients:
1 cup mushrooms
1 large celery stalk
1 clove garlic
1 to 2 tablespoons diced onion
1 1/2 teaspoons nama shoyu
1 1/2 teaspoons olive oil
2 tablespoons almonds
1 tablespoon ground golden flax
1/2 teaspoon sea salt
3/4 cup water (or more, depending on preference)
1 tablespoon nutritional yeast (optional)

Directions:
1) Place all of the ingredients except the water into a food processor or blender. Process or blend for a few seconds, then add the water slowly. Add more water if you want a thinner soup. *I think almond butter or tahini would make great substitutions for the almonds.

I'm sure this would be great with any nut or seed. Experiment! Source of recipe: I was playing around in the kitchen with some ingredients that I was left with towards the end of the week, and this was the result.

Raw Mushroom Stroganoff

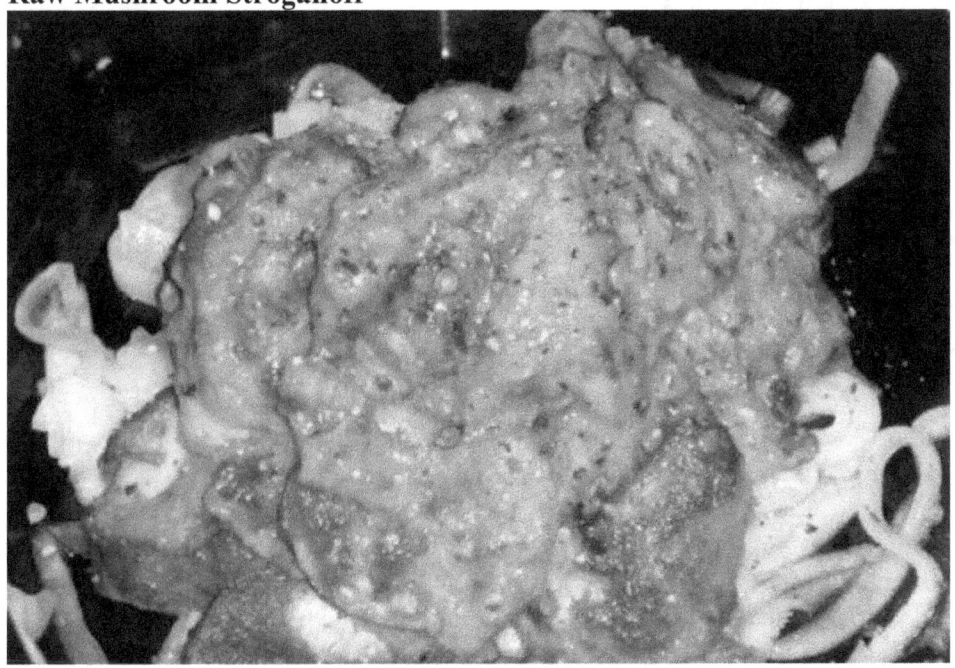

Preparation Time: 1 hour
Servings: 1-2

Ingredients:
3 cups baby portabellas, criminis mushrooms (either, or both)
1 cup water mushroom soak sauce for marinating:
1/4 cup water
1 tablespoon red onion
1 tablespoon olive oil
1 teaspoon braggs liquid aminos
1/4 teaspoon garlic powder

Stroganoff sauce:
1/2 cup almonds (soaked for 6 hours)
1 zucchini center (take out the seedy moist part of a zucchini)
1/4 teaspoon black pepper

1/4 teaspoon salt (optional)
1/2 teaspoon nutrional yeast
1/4 teaspoon paprika
1/4 teaspoon thyme
1-2 zucchinis or bag of kelp noodles, or shirataki noodles save the water from soaking the mushrooms

Directions:
First, soak your almonds, they take the longest. Next blend together the mushroom soak sauce together and mix in a bowl with 1/2 of the mushrooms. Let sit for 30-hour.

Soak the other mushrooms in the 1 cup of water with a splash of Braggs Liquid Aminos. After the almonds are soaked, blend or process them with 1/4 cup of the mushroom /soy water (not the sauce mix).

Then take a cheesecloth or a paper towel works too (if used gently), scrape almond mix into it, and gently squeeze the liquid out, it makes a creamy liquid. Save the almond pulp for something else, not this recipe. Now blend in the rest of the ingredients for your stroganoff sauce, with the mushrooms from the soy water mixture, until creamy. Take the mushrooms from the marinade, and place then on a non stick dehydrator sheet. Pour over them, the stroganoff sauce. Then drizzle 2 tablespoon of the marinate mixture over that. Dehydrate until warm, about 30-45 minutes. Serve over shredded or spiralized zucchini or kelp noodles, Its good with wild rice too (sprouted) but the flavors compete a little.

Raw Tahini Pad Thai

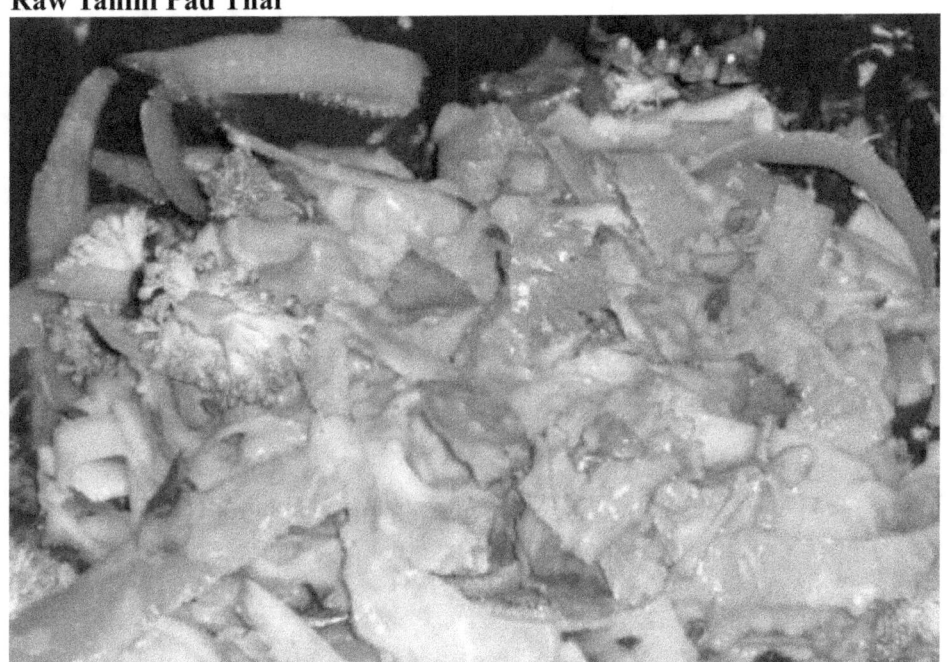

Preparation Time: 10 minutes
Servings: 1-2

Ingredients:
1 small or medium zucchini
sprinkle salt
1 large carrot
3 teaspoons raw tahini or almond butter
1 teaspoon vinegar (any kind except balsamic)
1 thumb sized piece ginger, chopped
1 clove garlic, chopped
3/4 teaspoon cayenne (or chili powder)
1 teaspoon Braggs Liquid Aminos
1 teaspoon dark miso
1-3 teaspoons water (depends on preference for thickness)
handful broccoli, chopped small

2 pinches cilantro mung bean or other sprouts, to serve

Directions:
1. Using a vegetable peeler (or spiralizer if you desire), peel the zucchini over and over until it's almost all peeled into strips, as much as you can. Chop up any leftover zucchini that you cannot peel into strips.

2. Sprinkle salt over this and set aside. The salt softens the zucchini. Repeat with the carrot but do not add salt. For sauce, add next 7 ingredients to blender (up to water).

3. You may have to scrape down the sides of your container to assist with blending. Add water, as desired, until you reach a consistency that you desire.

4. Squeeze the zucchini in your hands over a sink to drain the water. Place in bowl with carrots, add broccoli and toss. Pour sauce over these veggies. Top with sprouts and cilantro! Enjoy!

I love pad thai and peanut noodles! I just kind of put the same things I would in a pad Thai sauce, but without cooking. It came out great! It's definitely my new favorite raw meal!

That's Amore! Raw Pizza

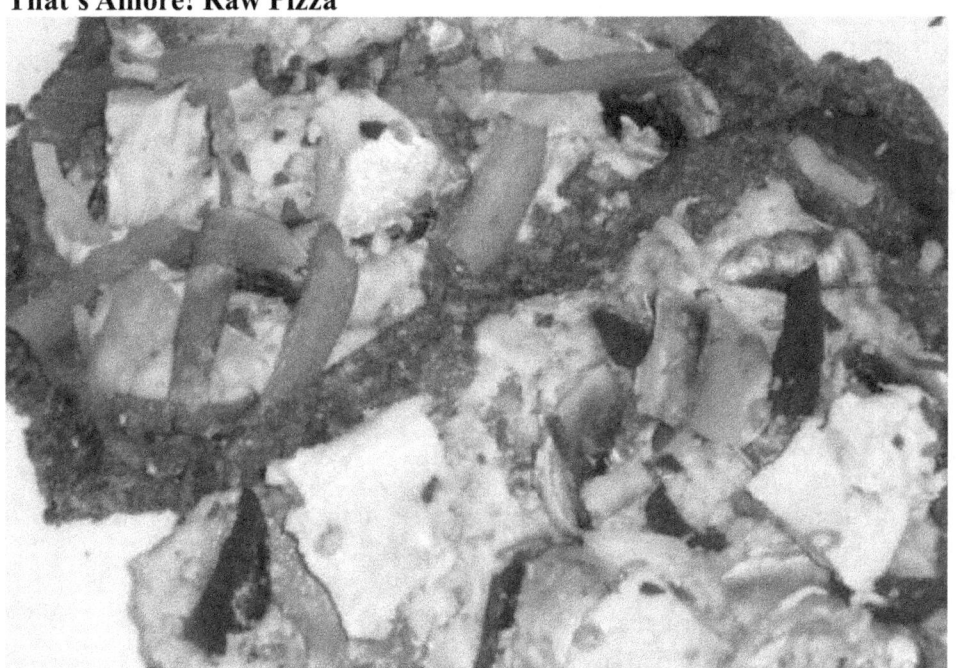

Preparation Time: 25 minutes
"Cooking" time: 6-9 hours Servings: 4

Ingredients:
1 cup sprouted rye
1/2 cup sprouted barley
1/2 cup sprouted spelt or oats (you can sub for any of the grains, whatever you have)
1/2 cup soaked sun dried tomatoes
1/4 cup onion
2 garlic cloves can add olives or carrots or red peppers if desired, easy to play with this.
1 teaspoon thyme
1 tablespoon basil
1 teaspoon oregano
pinch of salt and pepper

I like to add a little cayenne water as needed.

Directions:
Place all ingredients in processor. Grind up well, then slowly add water, grinding more, scraping often, until a paste is formed. Spread this onto non stick sheets (I use fruit roll up sheets that came with my dehydrator).

Spread evenly and pretty thick, about 3/4 inch, unless you want a really crisp crust. My dehydrator is big, so it only takes one tray for me. Time varies by dehydrator. It takes mine about 2 hours at 115, (AT THIS TIME SCORE A COUPLE SLICES OUT OF IT WITH KNIFE) then turn temp down to 105 and leave until dry to touch and able to easily! flip over with spatula. That takes about 2 more hours.

Once flipped, leave uniytl to your liking. I like mine crunchy on the edges, soft in the middle. Once done, be sure to store in the fridge in airtight container.

Pizza Sauce: 1/2 cup of soaked sundried tomatoes, water as needed, 1 tablespoon olive oil, pinch of thyme, pinch of salt, process Also! See recipe for raw cashew cheeze, It is great on pizza.

Add some lemon and nutritional yeast to it before spreading on pizza. Now put sauce and cheeze on your done pizza crust, add you fav toppings, like bell peppers (it really tastes like pizza with peppers and onions!!) mushrooms (soak for ten minutes first in salt water) etc. I personally really like beets on it! If you add avocado or pineapple, do that right before you eat.

Place the prepared pizza slices back in the dehydrator at 105- 115 (depending how long you wanna wait) and Voila! It's Amore! Remember you can sub ingredients, but the tomatoes and spices really help it to taste like pizza bread that you can even eat on your own. You can drop those ingredients if you want a plain tasting pizza crust.

Raw Zuppa di Pomodoro

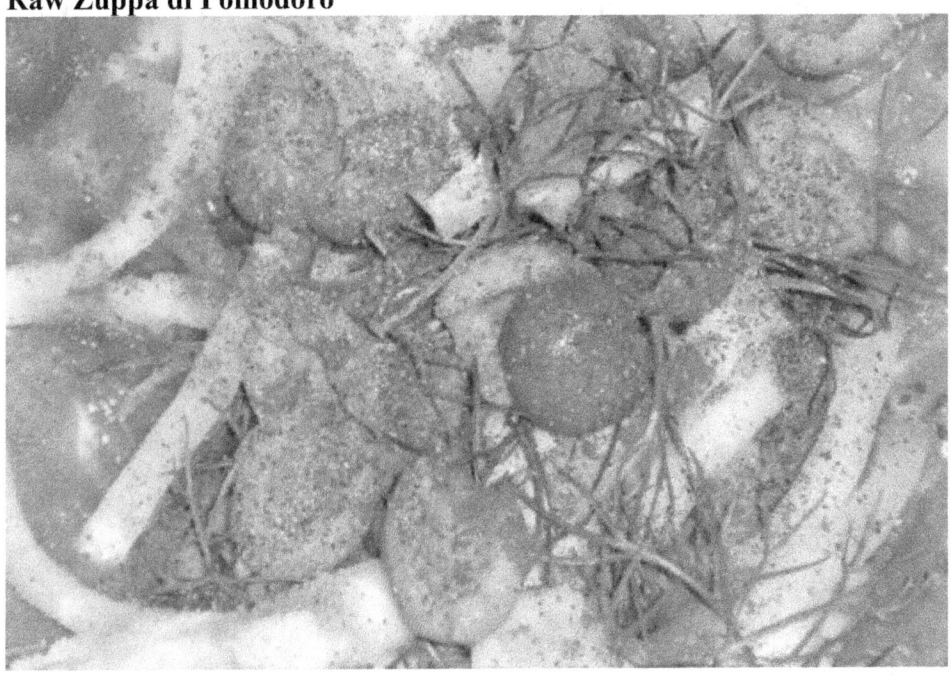

Preparation Time: 15 minutes
Servings: 1

Ingredients:
2 to 3 Roma tomatoes
2 teaspoons red wine vinegar or sherry
1 teaspoon jalapeno pepper
1 teaspoon red pepper
1 tablespoon olive oil
1 large tomato, diced
1/2 cup chopped olives
Salt and pepper, to taste

Directions:

1) Blend all ingredients except the diced tomatoes and olives until smooth. Pour into a bowl and garnish with diced tomato and olives. This makes a great plain tomato soup as well.

Incredible Raw Cabbage Rolls

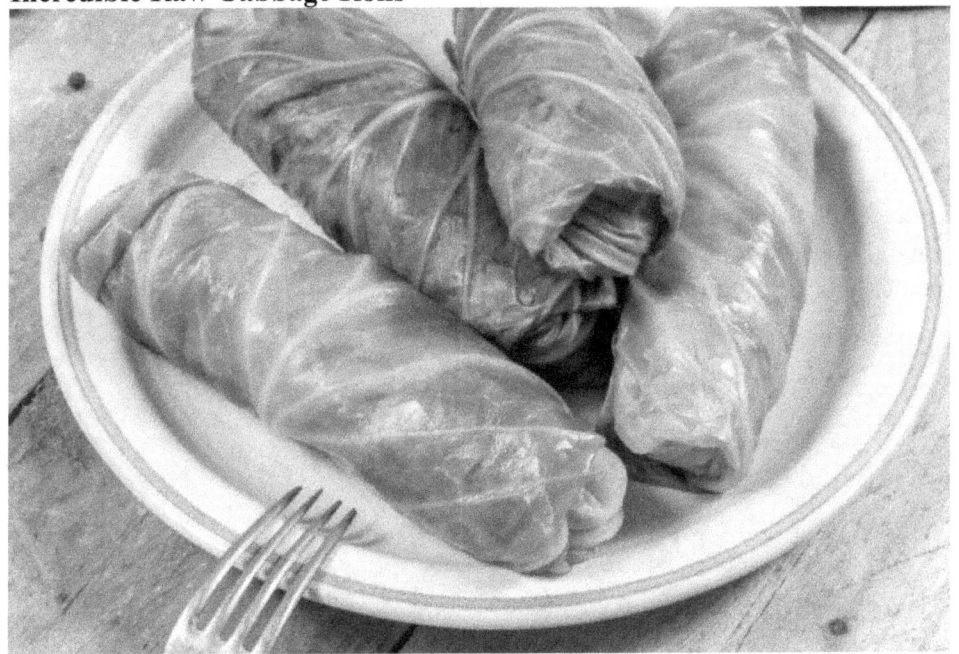

Preparation Time: 10 minutes

Ingredients:
8 cabbage leaves
1 red apple
1 stalk celery
2 carrots Cumin, pepper, and red pepper, to taste
2 scallions
2 cloves garlic
Zest of half a lime Juice of half a lime
1 tablespoon raw cider vinegar (maybe less)

Directions:
1) Pulse all ingredients but cabbage leaves in a food processor until finely chopped.

2) Remove the thickest part of cabbage stem by cutting a 'V' shape out of the bottom of each leaf. Place about 2 tablespoon of the mixture in the center of each leaf, squeezing lightly first remove excess drips. Roll up each leaf by folding in half away from you, then pulling the mixture tight against the wall you have created (closest to your body). Tuck in sides of leaf and continue to roll tightly.

3) Place the rolls seam side down on a platter and use toothpicks to hold in place if necessary. Serve with your favorite raw peanut sauce! Source of recipe: Modified from a recipe on 'Bean Vegan'.

Raw Curry

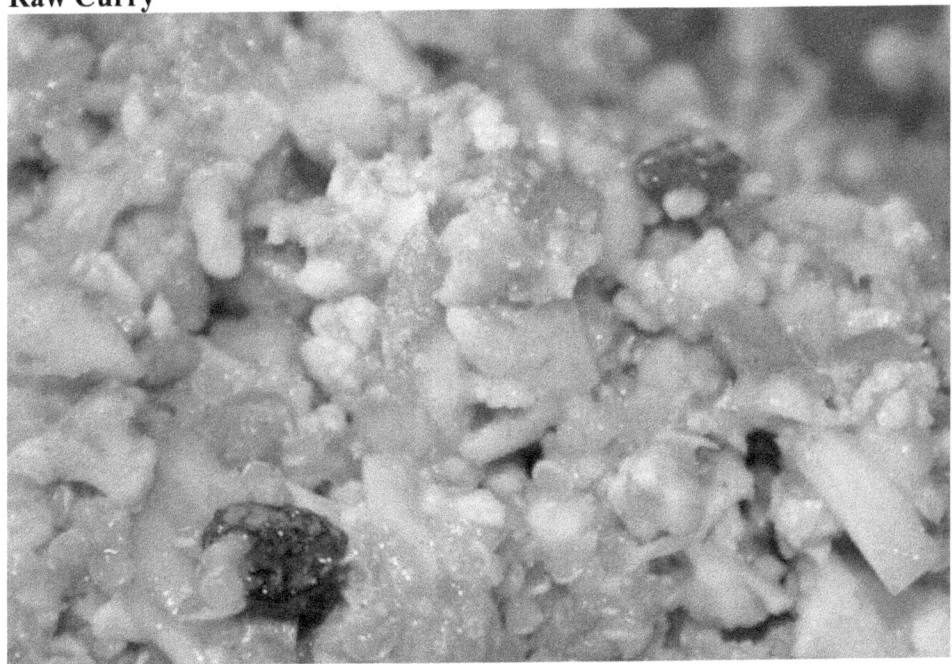

Preparation Time: 10 minutes
Servings: 2-3

Ingredients:
1-2 cups cauliflower cut in small pieces
1-2 carrots
1/2 onion Braggs Liquid Aminos
2-3 tablespoons raw tahini
raw curry powder
lemon juice
1 cup water cinnamon (optional)
raisins (optional)

Directions:
1. Cut or use food processor to make small pieces of the veggies.

2. In a separate bowl, combine the rest of the ingredients (except raisins if using)

3. Poor dressing slowly over veggies, stirring occasionally to coat everything. (Add the raisins here.)

4. Let marinate for at least 3 hours in the fridge.

5. Enjoy the deliciousness!

Rawritos!

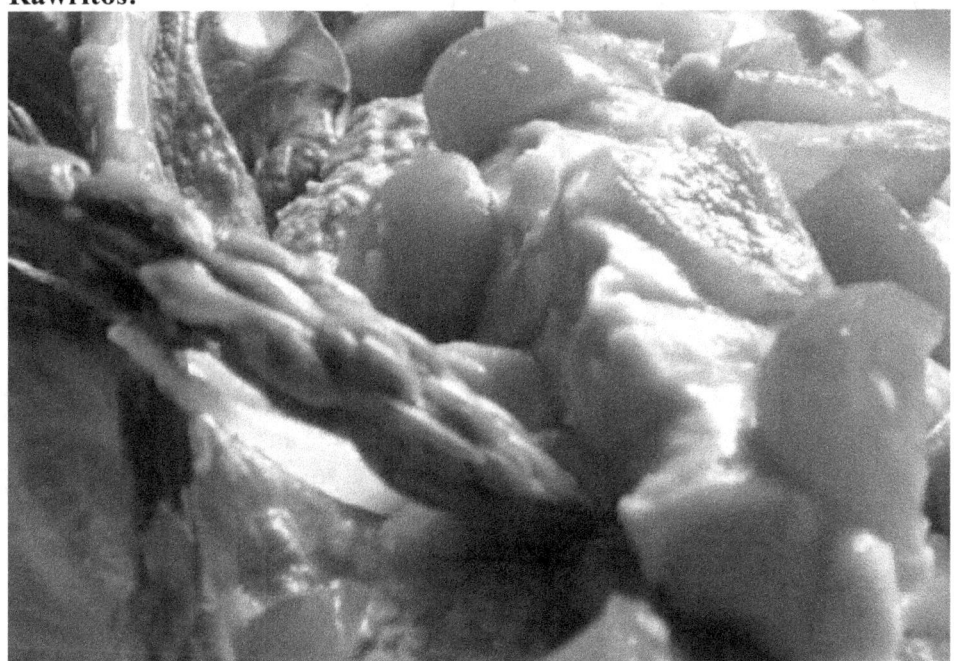

Preparation Time: 2 days
Servings: 1
Cooking Time: 5 minutes

Ingredients:
1 cup sprouted sunflower seeds (soaked overnight, sprout 1 day, use day after that. note: you can use sun seeds soaked for 4-8 hours)
1 teaspoon garlic powder
1 teaspoon chili powder
1 teaspoon cumin powder
1/2 teaspoon salt
sprinkle of cayenne (for extra spicyness)
1/2 teaspoon ground red pepper (optional)
1 teaspoon oil (olive)
1 teaspoon tahini
sprinkle of water

chopped tomatoes, onions, pickled jalepenos, whatever you like, I also used asparagus spears cashew sour cream (if desired)
large lettuce leaf.

Directions:
Now, I made this up today, so I just sprinkle here and there, but I'm pretty good at eye measuring. I added 1/2 teaspoon of everything first, processed, tasted, added another 1/2 of everything. Anyway!

So, taste as you go along and alter it as you wish! I tend to like a lot of spice and heat! These are a really wonderful substitute for refried beans! They taste awesome!

Okay, Process together everything except the lettuce and condiments. Depending on your food processor, you may need to add a sprinkle of water. It won't be completely smooth, kinda beany looking. Spoon down the middle of the lettuce, add toppings and fold over the sides of the lettuce while you eat!! Enjoy!

Eccentric Raw Sushi

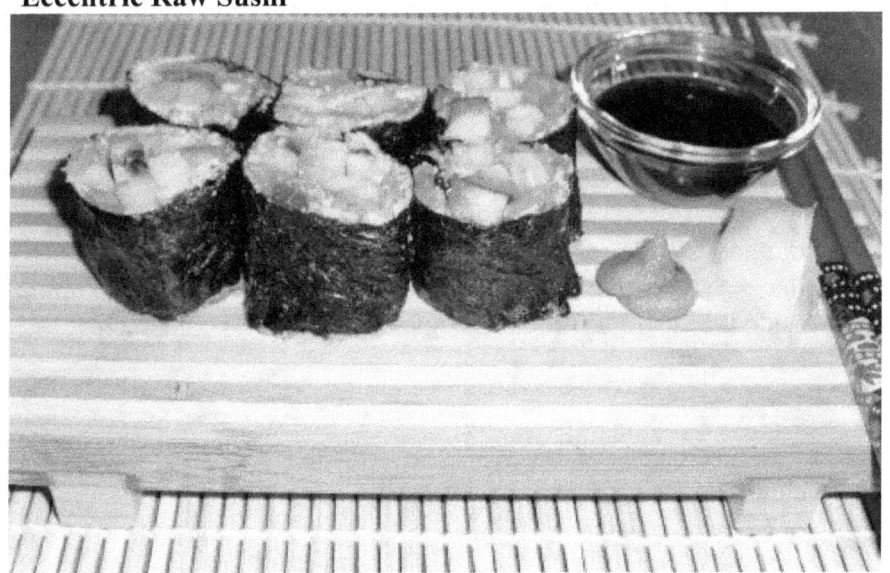

Preparation Time: 20 minutes
Servings: 6

Ingredients:
6 nori sheets, not roasted
5 carrots, grated finely
1 cup miscellaneous sushi veggies, grated finely (I like radishes, cucumber, peppers, green onions, mushrooms)
1 cup sprouts, chopped fresh horseradish or wasabi, grated, optional
1/4 cup Bragg's liquid aminos, for dipping

Directions:
1. Take nori seaweed sheets and lay carrots on top (as you would normally with sushi rice), leaving a space at each lateral end of the nori sheets.

2. Place veggies and sprouts in 1 of the spaces on the nori paper and sprinkle with grated horseradish or wasabi, if using.

3. Roll up the nori sheets, making the veggies in the center of your roll. Wet the end of nori sheet with Bragg's or water to help it stay in place.

4. With a very sharp knife, slice roll into little sushi sections which can be dipped in Bragg's or whatever dip of your choice and enjoy. Viola! You have raw sushi! A tiny bit of grated ginger mixed in with the grated carrot gives quite a nice zing.

Make sure your hands and preparation area are dry when assembling the sushi. If you have a sweet tooth, try sliced mango, banana, or shredded apple and raisins inside the sushi in place of veggies. Hope you like the recipe.

Raw Tacos

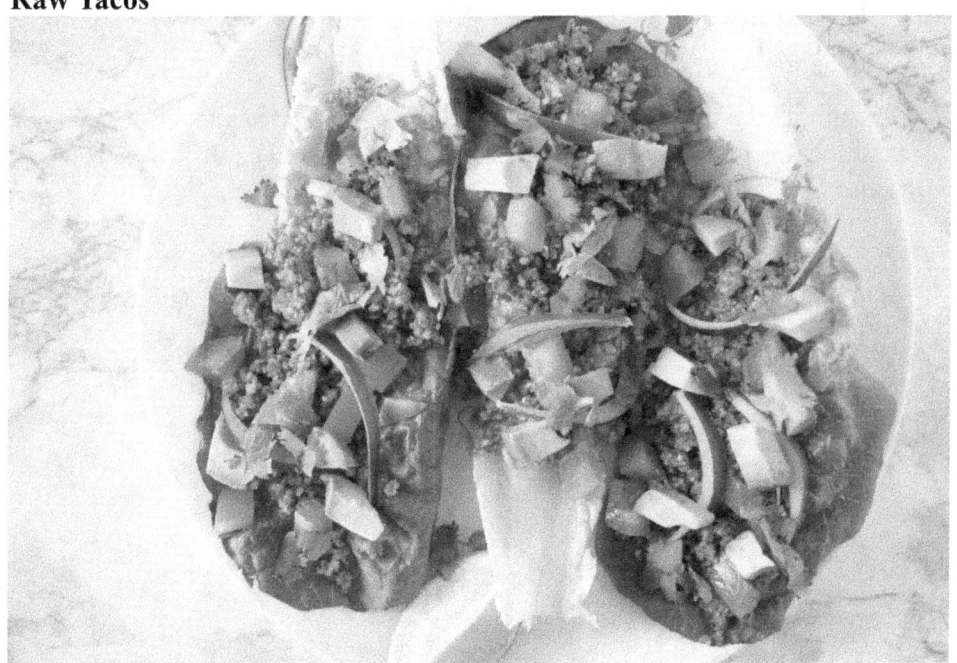

Preparation Time: 15 minutes
Servings: 3

Ingredients:
1/2 avocado
3 slices green pepper
1 slice onion
Lemon juice
Garlic powder
Salt
3 pieces romaine, green leaf, or red leaf lettuce
Pico de gallo salsa, as desired
2 slices each red and yellow pepper
1/2 cup broccoli and cauliflower florets

Directions:

1) Mash the avocado in a bowl. Chop 1 slice of green pepper and half the onion slice and add to the avocado. Season to taste with lemon juice, garlic powder, and salt, thus making raw guacamole.

2) To assemble, lay down a leaf of lettuce and spread with a layer of guacamole. Top with pico, peppers, onion, broccoli, and cauliflower. Top with salsa and fold in the back and roll up sides.

Samosa (raw vegan)

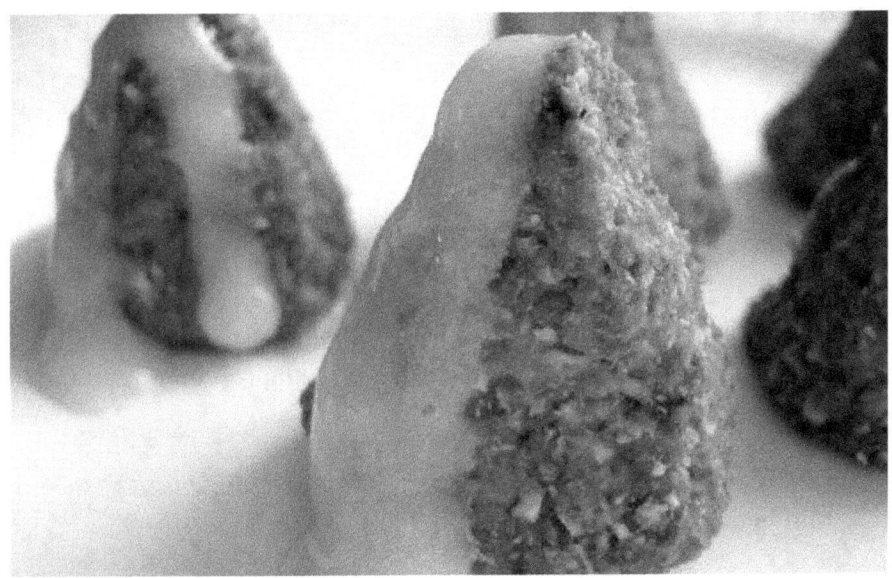

Preparation Time: 20-30 minutes
Servings: 4

Ingredients:
1 head cauliflower, chopped
1 yam, chopped
1 zucchini, chopped
1/4 cup walnuts
1/4 cup raisins
2 dates
2 cloves garlic, pressed
1 cup green peas
juice of 1 lemon
4 tablespoons olive oil
1 tablespoon curry powder
1 teaspoon cumin

1 teaspoon red pepper flakes
1 teaspoon salt
1 medium onion, finely minced
2 jalapeno, finely minced

Mango sauce:
1 mango, peeled and chopped
3 tablespoons agave
1/2 cup water

Directions:
1. In a food processor with an "S" blade, process the cauliflower, yam, zucchini, walnuts, raisins, dates, and garlic until pureed. This is a lot and I processed this in a few batches. Mix together with the rest of the samosa ingredients.

2. Form into cone shapes or triangular patties and dehydrate for several hours, until the outside is a bit crispy but the inside is still soft.

3. To make the mango sauce, simply puree mango with the agave and water until smooth. Serve the samosas with a generous dollop of mango sauce.

4 servings 2 1/2 per serving

Raw Jamacian Shishkabobs

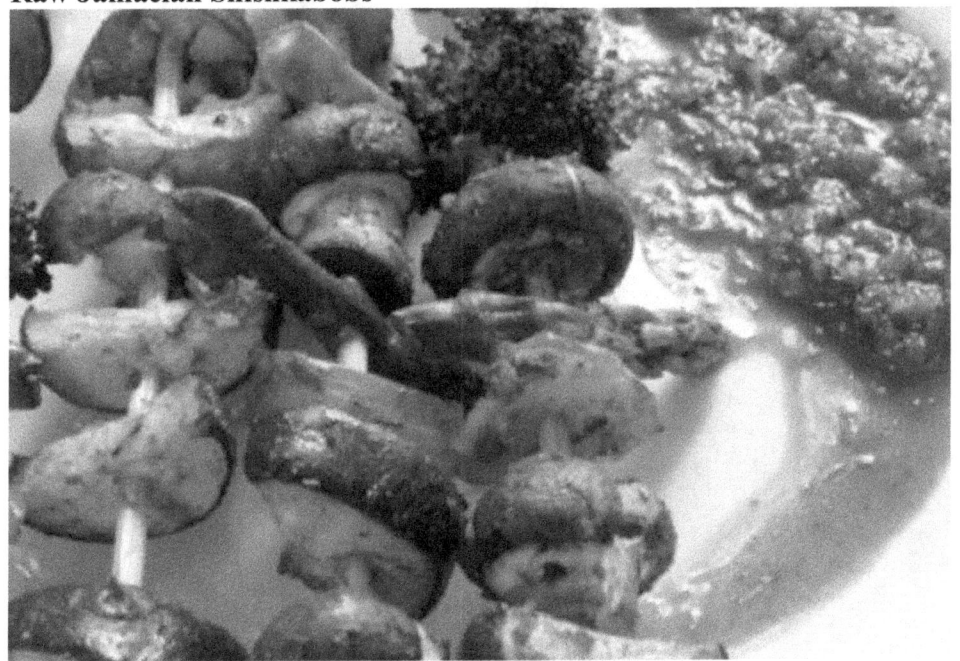

Preparation Time: 10 minutes
"Cooking" time: 2 hours Servings: 2-4

Ingredients:
3/4 teaspoon allspice
1/4 teaspoon nutmeg
1/2 teaspoon thyme
1/8 teaspoon cinnamon
1/8 teaspoon cayenne
1/8 teaspoon ground ginger (or fresh)
1/4 teaspoon red pepper
1/4 teaspoon black pepper
1/2 habanero or jalapeno
1 clove garlic
1/4 chopped onion
1 tablespoon olive oil

1 tablespoon agave
1/2 tablespoon Braggs Liquid Aminos
1 lemon wedge, squeezed
zucchini, broccoli, red peppers, baby portabellas, grape tomatoes, asparagus, you pick veggies skewers

Directions:
1) Blend all of the ingredients except vegetables.

2) Marinate vegetables at least 20 min in this sauce.

3) Skewer the vegetables and place on dehydrator and dry for 2 hours to warm.

Garlic and Chive Mashed No-tatoes

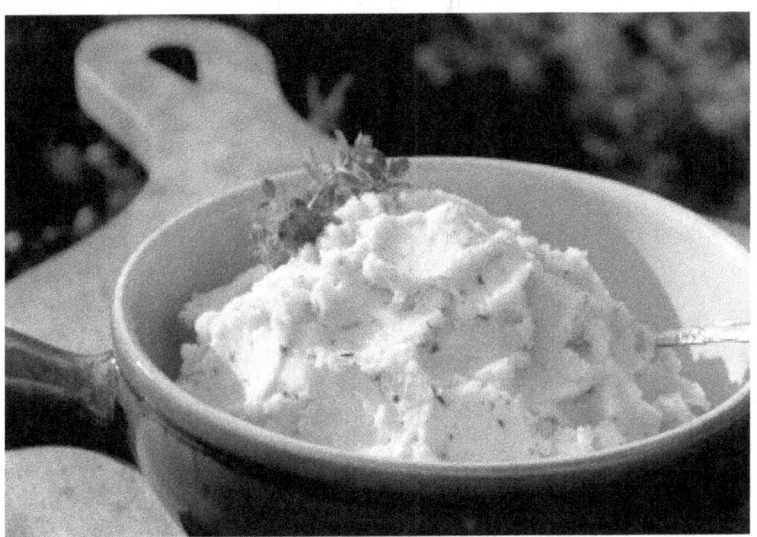

These garlic and chive mashed no-tatoes are simply amazing. They are easy to make and absolutely delicious. Every mouthful is creamy, rich and oh, so heavenly. No need to wait until the holidays to have the perfect comfort food. These are great any time of year!

Ingredients
2 1/4 cups celery root, peeled and chopped
3/4 cup cashews
1 Tbs white miso paste
1 tsp onion powder
2 tsp nutritional yeast
1 1/4 tsp Himalayan pink salt
1/2 cup Irish moss paste
3/4 cup water (add more if necessary for creamy texture)
1 Tbs garlic, minced
1/4 tsp white pepper
1Tbs chives, minced

Instructions

1. Add all ingredients (except chives) into blender and blend on high until creamy and warm.

2. Blend chives in by hand, then serve.

3. These No-tatoes can be served warm by blending in your blender. Another way is to place them in the dehydrator for 1 hour.

Raw Vegan Spinach Manicotti

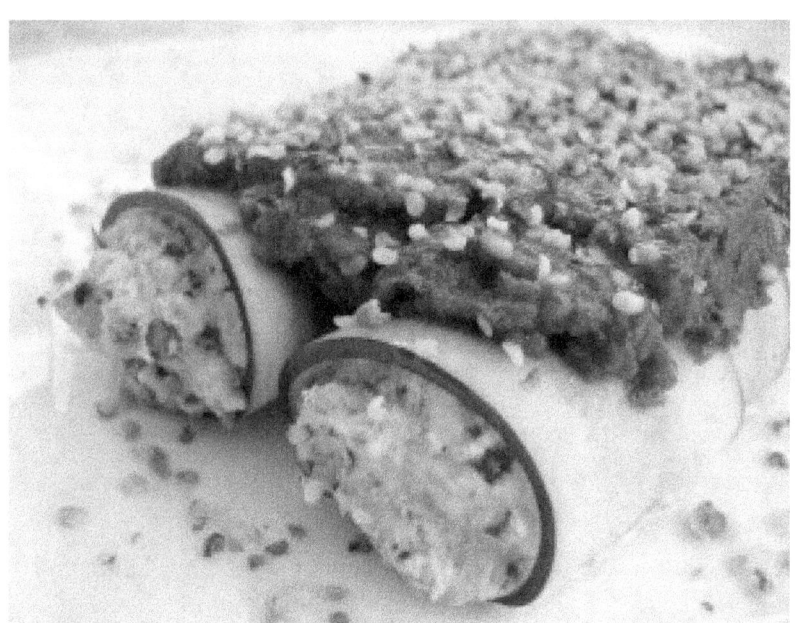

Ingredients:
For the Noodles:
4 medium zucchini
2 tablespoons olive oil

For the Spinach & Sunflower Cheese Filling:
2 cups of sunflower seeds (from above)
½ cup water
½ cup lemon juice
3 cloves of garlic
1 teaspoon Himalayan salt
8 cups spinach
½ cup parsley
1½ tablespoons Italian Seasoning

For the Herby Tomato Sauce:
3 cups of sundried tomatoes, measured after soaking (from above)
1 cup water
1 medium tomato, chopped
¼ cup cold-pressed olive oil
3 cloves of garlic
1 tablespoon oregano
1 tablespoon basil
2 teaspoons rosemary
2 teaspoons thyme
1 teaspoon fennel seed
½-1 teaspoon salt, only if your sun-dried tomatoes are unsalted
2 tablespoons hemp seed, for garnish, if desired

Instructions:
Advanced Prep

1. Soak 2 cups of sunflower seeds in pure water for 4-6 hours. Drain and rinse.

2. In a separate bowl, soak 2 cups of sundried tomatoes in pure water for 4 hours or longer. Drain

For the Noodles

1. Cut off both ends of each zucchini. Using a mandoline, slice the zucchini the long way so that you have long, wide noodles. If a mandoline is not available, use a knife, cutting as thinly as possible.

2. Place in a bowl, drizzle with olive oil and toss very gently.

For the Spinach & Sunflower Cheese Filling

1. In a high-speed blender, combine sunflower seeds, water, lemon, garlic and salt.

2. Blend well until smooth. Scrape into a large bowl.

3. In a food processor, process the spinach and parsley in batches until chopped but not puréed. Alternately, chop finely by hand. Pour into the bowl with the sunflower cheese.

4. Add Italian seasoning and mix well.

For the Herby Tomato Sauce

1. To assemble, arrange 4 zucchini noodles horizontally on a cutting board, slightly overlapping one over the next by about ½".

2. Place ¼ cup of the spinach & sunflower cheese filling in the center and spread so that it covers the front to the back and about 1" in width.

3. Roll the zucchini from left to right to create a filled manicotti.

4. Place two manicotti on a plate and top with ¼ cup of tomato sauce.

5. Garnish with a drizzle of olive oil and a sprinkling of hemp seeds and/or Italian seasoning.

Rawesome Tom Yum Spicy Thai Soup

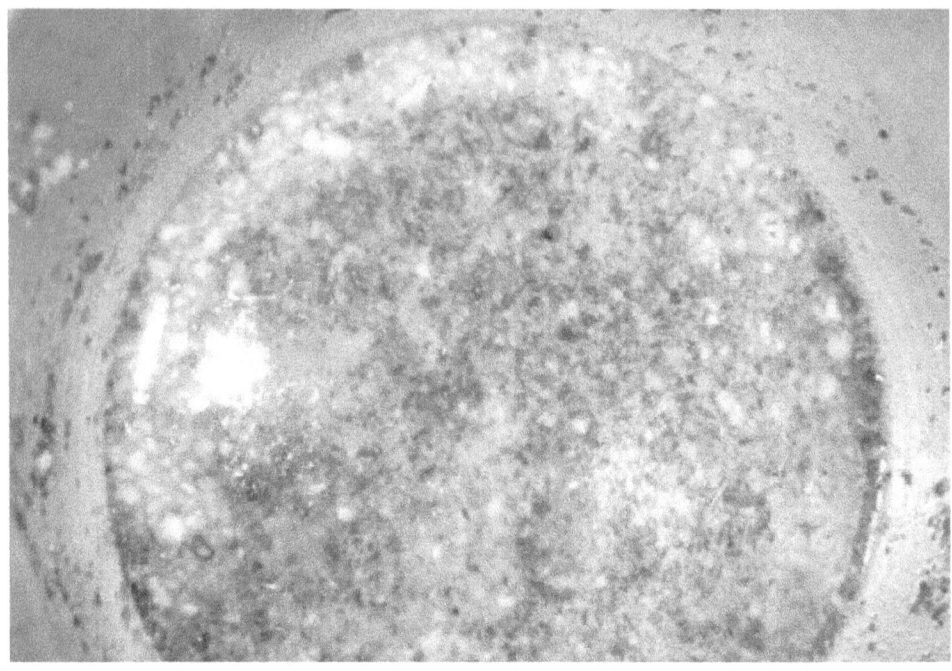

Preparation Time: 10 minutes
Servings: 1

Ingredients:
1/2 cup coconut meat
1/2 coconut water
1/4 to 1 whole jalapeno or Serrano pepper
1 good pinch oregano
Pinch basil

Directions:
1) Warm a heat-proof bowl in the oven for ten minutes to warm.

2) Combine all ingredients in a blender and blend until smooth. Pour into warmed bowl. SO good! This is sure to warm you up on a cold day and clear

your sinuses. It sounds too simple, but the sweetness of the coconut and the spicy warmth of the peppers is divine.

Raw Carrot Falafel with Creamy Tahini Sauce

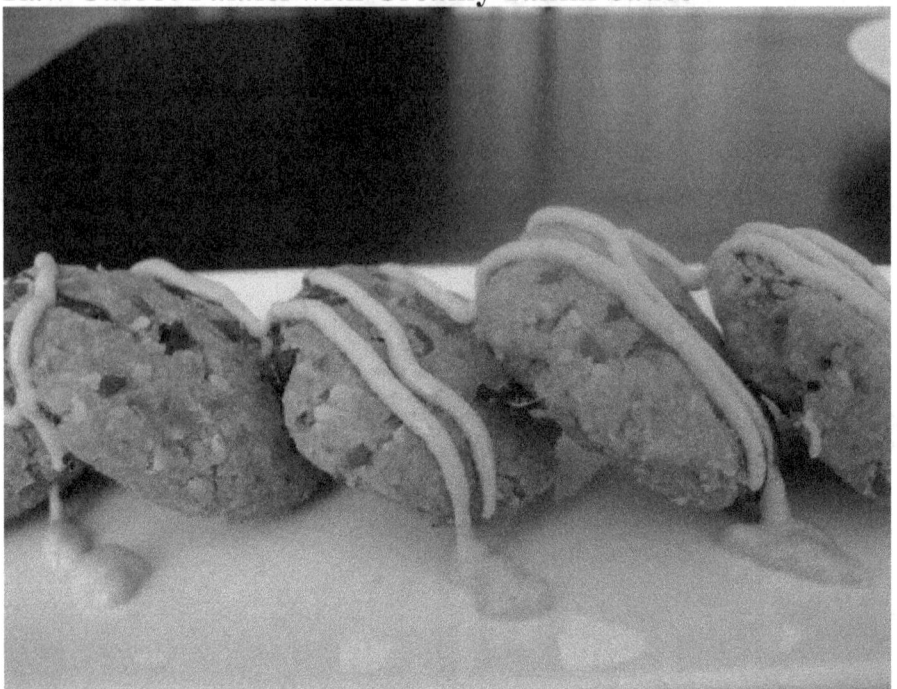

Carrot pulp, ground sesame seeds and flax, fresh herbs and spices all rolled up into yummy little falafel patties! To acquire your carrot pulp simply make a large batch of carrot juice and enjoy. This is actually a nut-free recipe and the base of carrot pulp really makes this recipe a lot easier on the digestive system. The tahini sauce is super creamy and tangy and makes a delicious salad dressing in its own right.

Ingredients:
For the Falafel
2 cups carrot pulp
1 cup sesame seeds, ground in a coffee or spice grinder, a magic bullet, or a food processor
2 tbsp ground flax seed
1 tsp salt
1 tbsp lemon juice
2 1/2 tbsp olive oil
1 stalk celery, finely chopped

1/4 cup Italian flat leaf parsley, chopped
1/4 cup cilantro, chopped
1 clove garlic, minced very finely (optional)
1/4 cup onion, minced finely (optional)

Tangy Tahini Sauce (makes about 1 1/2 cups)
1/4 cup tahini
1 tbsp lemon juice
2 tbsp water
1 tbsp apple cider vinegar
1 tbsp agave syrup or 1/2 packet stevia
1/2 tsp cumin
1/2 tsp coriander
2 tbsp nama shoyu
1/2 large or 1 very small clove garlic, minced (optional)

Instructions:
For the Falafel:

1) Mix all ingredients very well by hand, as if you were making meatloaf.

2) Roll into balls about 1 1/2-2 inches thick, flatten gently, and put on a dehydrator try lined with a Paraflex sheet OR onto a baking sheet.

3) Dehydrate the falafel at 115 degrees for two hours.

4) Remove the Paraflex sheet, flip them over, and dehydrate for another two hours.

If using an oven, bake them at 175 degrees with the oven door ajar for an hour and repeat on the other side.

Tangy Tahini Sauce:

1) Blend all ingredients in a magic bullet, VitaMix, blender, or food processor until smooth and creamy. The sauce should be super tangy and delicious!

Assembly

Simply plate a few of these, drizzle them with sauce, and serve. The sweet, nutty, spicy quality of the falafel is balanced by the acidity of the tahini sauce. In all? An awesome raw take on a Middle Eastern classic.

Swamp Soup (a.k.a. Green Gazpacho)

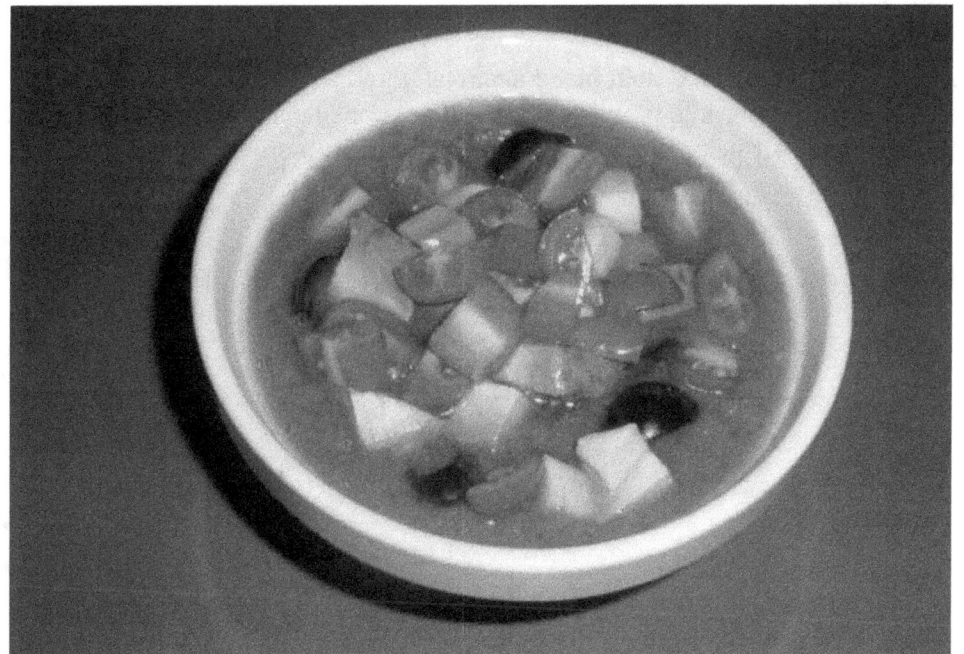

Preparation Time: 15 minutes
Servings: 3 to 4

Ingredients:
4 large tomatoes, peeled and chopped
1/2 large cucumber, peeled and chopped
1/2 bell pepper, seeded and chopped
1/2 small onion, chopped
1 clove garlic, pressed
1/2 jalapeno pepper, diced
1 to 2 kale leaves, torn into pieces
Juice of 1/2 large lemon
Celtic sea salt, to taste Avocado, diced (optional)
Green onions, sliced (optional)

Directions:
1) Place tomatoes, cucumber, bell pepper, onion, garlic, jalapeño, kale, lemon juice and salt into the pitcher of a blender or food processor and blend until smooth.

2) Chill for 2 hours and then blend again as liquid will separate some. To serve as soup, pour into bowls and top with chopped avocado and sliced green onions. Or just drink it like a smoothie! Turns a brownish green that looks a bit like swamp muck, hence the name.

Sweet Potato Pasta with Tangy Marinara: a Raw Food Recipe

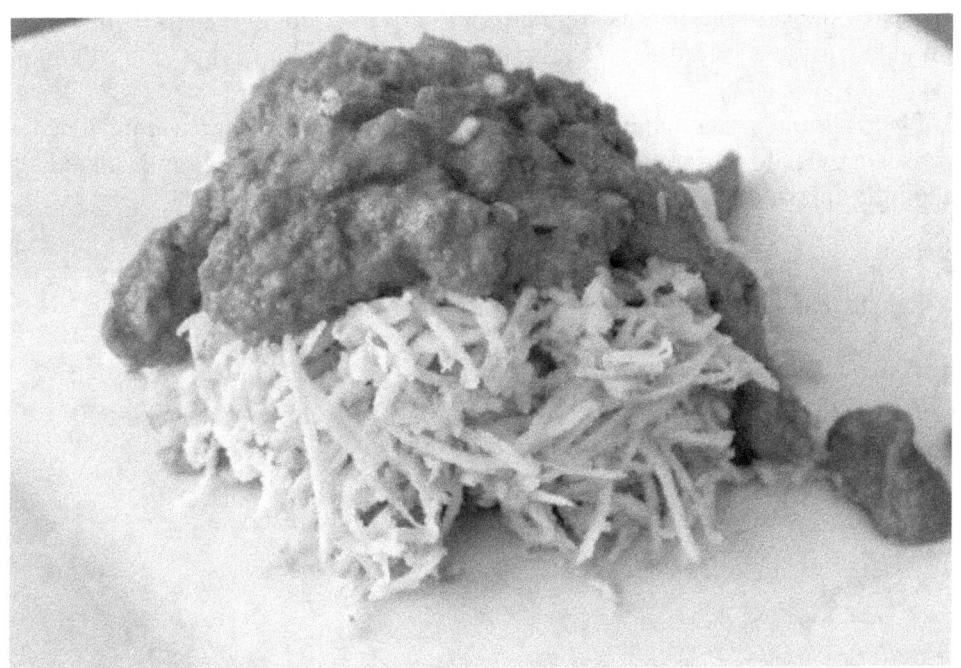

Ingredients:
7 sun-dried tomato halves
1/4 cup raw almonds, soaked
2-4 hours and dried
1 teaspoon lemon juice
1 teaspoon olive oil
1/2 teaspoon oregano
1/2 teaspoon basil
1/2 teaspoon salt
dash red pepper flakes
1 sweet potato
2 roma tomatoes, chopped.

Directions:

1. Place sun-dried tomatoes in bowl of warm water to start softening. Set aside. (Raw foodists take care not to use water hotter than 118 degrees F.)

2. I leave the skin on the sweet potato. Shred it into lengthy strips using the small side of a standard shredder or spiralizer. Set aside.

3. Place almonds in a blender or food processor and blend into a flour-like consistency. Add lemon juice, olive oil, and seasonings. Blend until mixed, adding a splash of water as necessary.

4. Chop sun-dried tomatoes and add to the sauce base, along with roma tomatoes. Blend into a thick, creamy marinara sauce.

5. Divide sweet potato noodles into 2 servings and top with tangy marinara sauce. Garnish with additional red pepper flakes, if you wish. Sauce will keep in the fridge for two days.

Raw! Raw! Teriyaki Veggies with Wild Rice

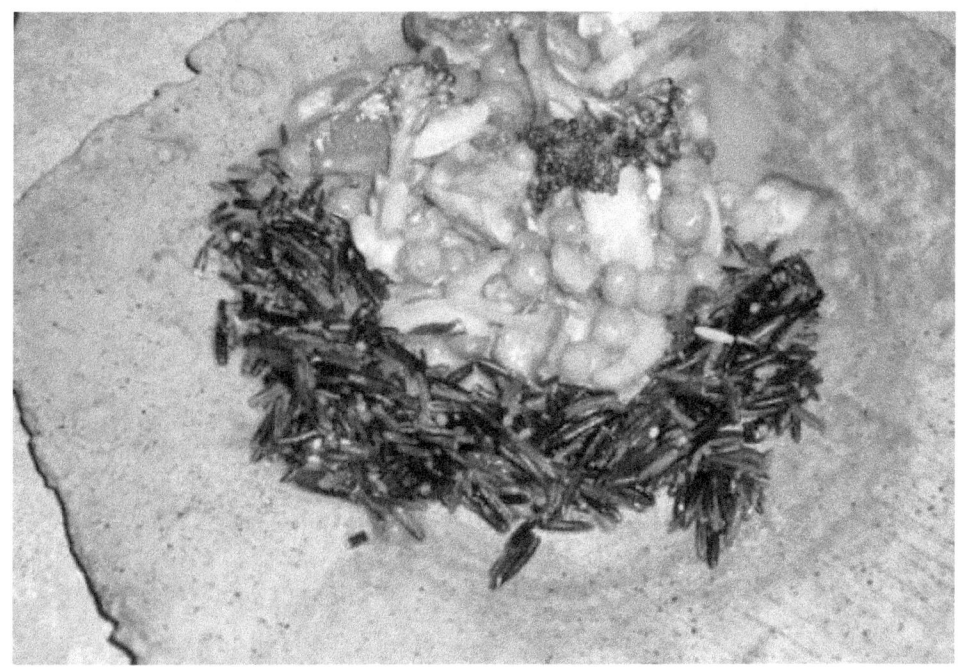

Preparation Time: 1 day 15 minutes
"Cooking' time: 5 minutes
Servings: 1-2

Ingredients:
Vegetables and rice:
1/2 cup wild rice stir fry mixture (I use broccoli, napa cabbage, red and green peppers, mushrooms, zucchini, peas, onions), chopped

Sauce:
2 tablespoons Braggs Liquids Aminos (raw transition food)
1 tablespoon olive oil
2 teaspoons agave nectar (substitute, if desired)
1 garlic clove
1/2" piece ginger

1 teaspoon lemon juice (3 teaspoons orange juice for "orange chicken" flavor).

Directions:

1. Place rice in bowl, and fill bowl with water to cover the rice. Let soak over night. Rinse in the morning, soak again for 4-5 hours, rinse again. It should now be soft to the bite.

2. If not soft to your liking, soak another 5 hours, then rinse and let air dry while you make the rest of your dinner. I have done this cycle for up to four days and the rice is still good. It has this wonderful earthy smell. I like mine a tad chewy.

3. Now place all sauce ingredients into food processor and process. Place vegetables in a bowl, and pour sauce on top; mix. You can now place rice on a plate and top with veggies, or 4. Pour the veggies with sauce on to a nonstick sheet for your dehydrator and dehydrate at 110 degrees F for 5-10 minutes. This really helps the veggies to soak a little flavor in and soften a tiny bit. When done, just pour onto rice and enjoy!! This is a great recipe for someone who has never tried raw, or someone you are trying to convince that it is not all salads.

Raw Tomato "Pasta"

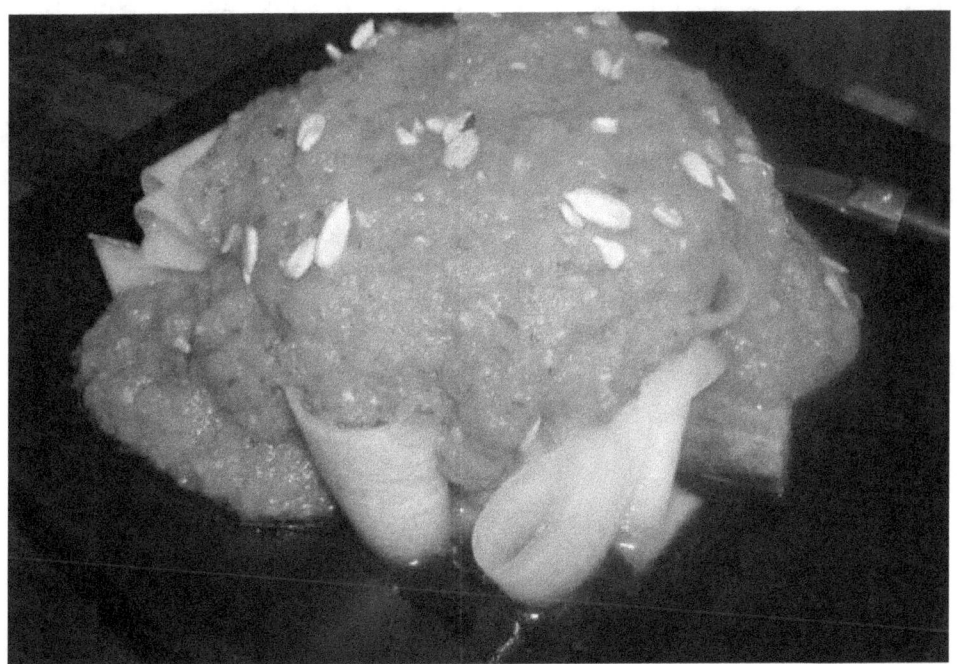

Preparation Time: 1 to 5 minutes
Servings: 1

Ingredients:
1 medium-large tomato
1 cucumber (6 to 7 inches, not too thick)
1 tablespoon FRESH dill, or to taste
1/2 tablespoon fresh thyme, or to taste
1 garlic clove
1 teaspoon oil
1 teaspoon dry parsley (or 1 tablespoon fresh)
1/2 spring onion
Sunflower seeds for topping (optional)
Salt & pepper, to taste.

Directions:

1) Peel your cucumber. Slice it into noodle like shapes, I used a potato peeler and shaved mine, it turned out like fresh fettuccine. Put your "noodles" in a strainer or on-top of a kitchen towel to absorb some of the moisture, this isn't required but your pasta will be soupy if not.

2) In a blender add tomato, I don't seed mine, but I do take out the stem area. Pulse that for a few seconds. Add the rest of the ingredients and blend until smooth, or until your desired consistency.

3) Toss sauce with "noodles" or pile sauce on top. Sprinkle on some raw sunflower seeds for extra crunch. This recipe is super quick--only took me 2 minutes!

Mushroom "Bul Go Gi"

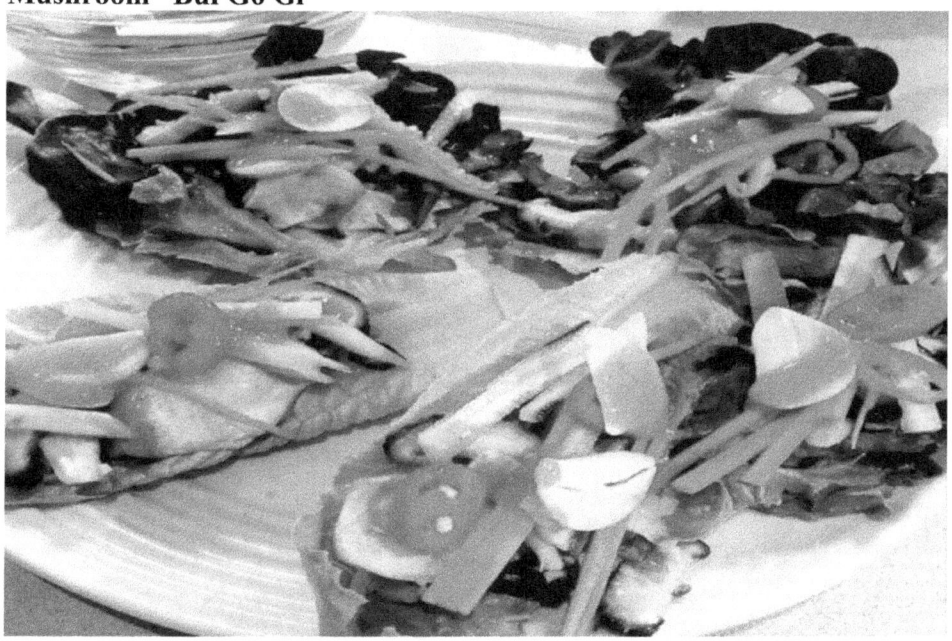

Ingredients:
- 4 cups sliced mushrooms
- 2 tablespoons tamari
- 1 tablespoon toasted sesame oil
- 1/2 tablespoon minced garlic
- 1/2 cup Asian pear, micro-planes or pureed in food processor

Fillings:
- 1 clove thinly sliced mushroom
- 1 Korean or jalapeño pepper, sliced
- 1 cup julienned cucumber
- 1 cup julienned carrot

Wrappers:
- 8 red lettuce leaves or more

Gochujang Sauce:

- 2 1/2 tablespoons unpasteurized miso, any color
- 2 tablespoons toasted sesame oil
- 1/4 cup agave syrup or coconut nectar
- 1/2 teaspoon chili powder or cayenne (to taste)

Instructions:

1. Toss together all BulGoGi ingredients in one bowl. Set aside to marinate for 15 minutes, until softened.

2. Prepare fillings, and set aside.

3. Squeeze excess marinade from mushrooms, and place into each lettuce leaf. Top with fillings.

4. Whisk Gochujang ingredients to mix well, and drizzle on top of lettuce wraps.

Peanut Noodles

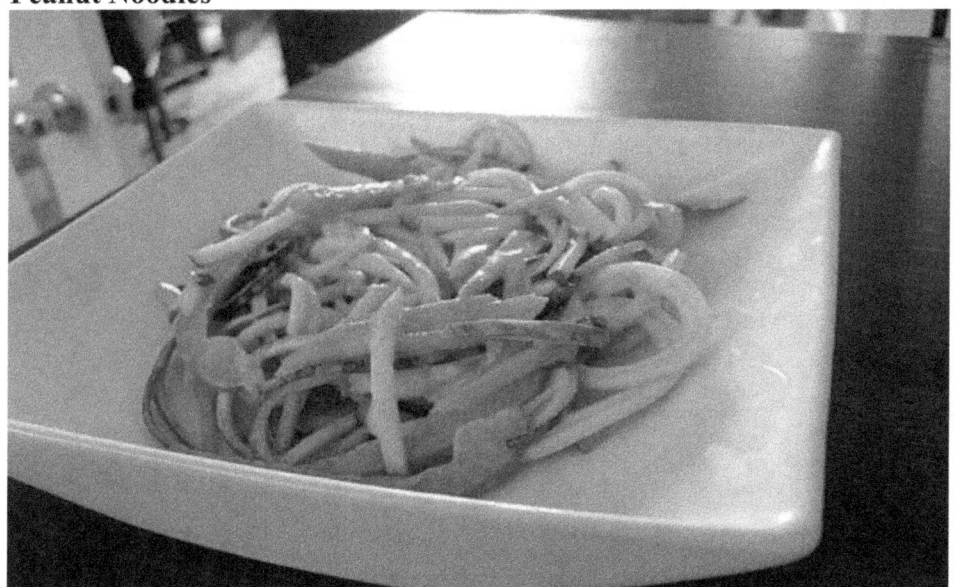

Ingredients:

Peanut Sauce:
- 1 inch ginger
- 1 cup olive oil (or flax oil)
- 2 teaspoons sesame oil
- Juice of 1 lime • 4 tablespoons mellow white miso
- 6 dates, pitted OR 1/4 cup agave
- 2 tablespoons nama shoyu
- 1/3 cup water

Noodles:
- 1 large or 2 small zucchinis, spiralized or sliced with a vegetable peeler
- 1/2 red pepper, sliced into matchsticks
- 1/2 carrot, sliced into matchsticks
- 1/4 large or 1/2 small cucumber, grated or peeled into long strips
- Scallions or green onions to garnish

Instructions:

1. Blend all sauce ingredients till creamy and emulsified.

2. Prepare and mix all veggies, save the scallions or green onion.

3. Toss with 1/4 cup sauce, adding more if necessary, and sprinkle with scallions.

Notes Add sugar snaps, shitake mushrooms, snow pea shoots, or mung bean sprouts for an extra crunch!

Spicy Tacos with Nacho Cheeze

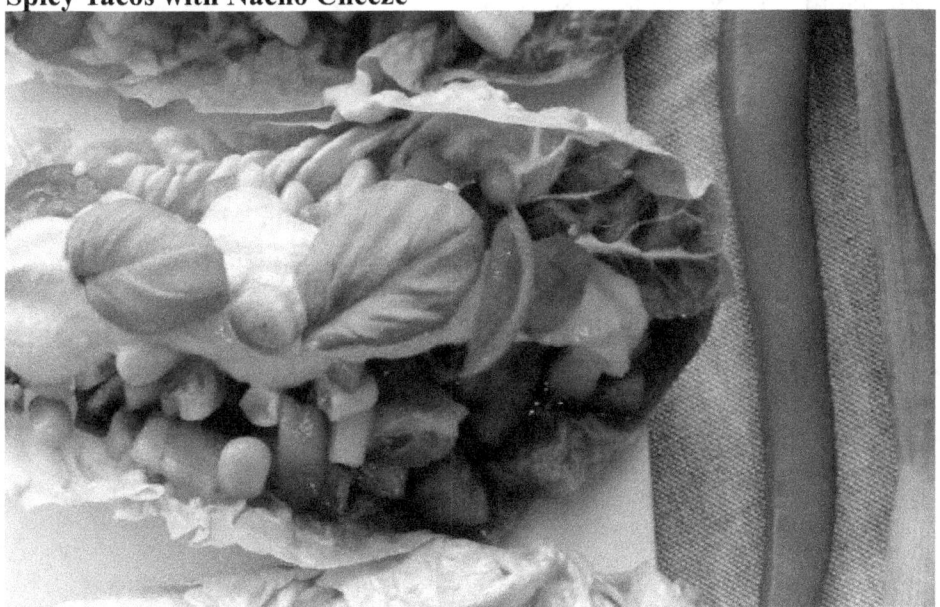

Ingredients:
- 2 small heads of romaine lettuce
- 1 diced English cucumber
- 2 cups cherry tomatoes, diced
- 2 red bell peppers, diced
- 1 cup white mushrooms, diced
- 1 bunch green onion, diced
- 1 medium red onion, diced
- 1/2 cup organic raw corn
- 1/2 jalapeno chili
- Juice of 1 lemon
- 1/2 teaspoon paprika
- 1/2 teaspoon Himalayan pink crystal salt

Nacho cheeze:
- 1 cup raw cashews, soaked overnight
- 1 red bell pepper, diced
- 1/2 medium red onion, diced

- 1/2 teaspoon turmeric
- Pinch of Himalayan pink crystal salt
- Juice of 1/2 lemon
- 2 tablespoons water

Instructions:
1. For the tacos, mix diced cucumber, tomatoes, bell pepper, mushrooms, onions, and corn. In a small bowl, whisk together lemon juice, paprika powder, sea salt and jalapenos and pour over mixed veggies. Let marinate for 30 minutes at room temperature.

2. For the nacho cheeze, blend nuts with bell pepper, onion, turmeric, sea salt, lemon juice, and water.

3. Fill mixed spicy veggies into romaine leaves and top with nacho cheeze.

Veggie Burger with Sunflower Bread

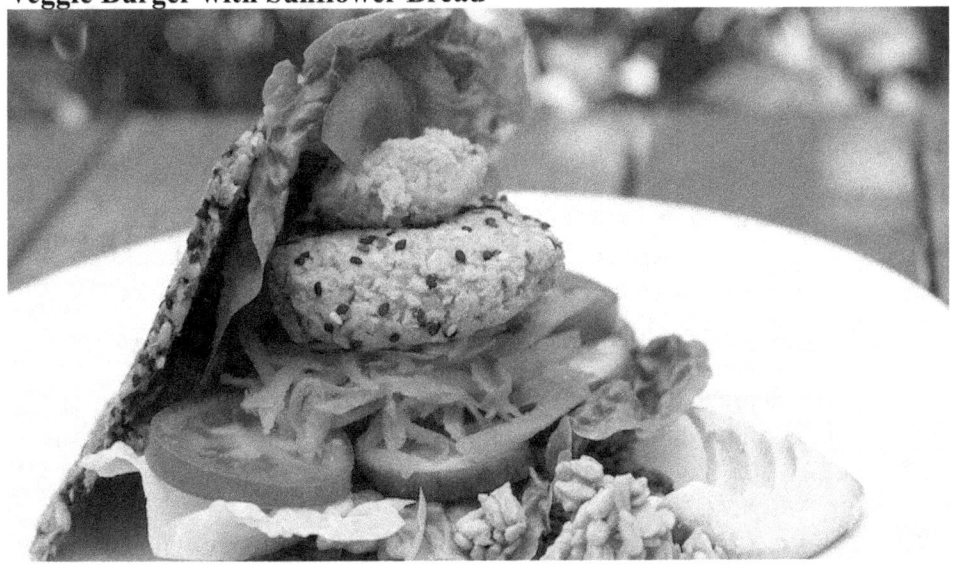

Ingredients:

Quick and Tasty Raw Sunflower Seed Bread:
- 1 cup of ground flaxseeds
- 1/3 cup of whole flaxseeds
- ½ teaspoon of salt
- 2 tablespoons of finely chopped celery
- 1 cup of water
- 1/3 cup of tamari
- 2/3 cup of sunflower seeds
- ¼ cup of black sesame seeds

Chickpea Burgers:
- 4 cups of sprouted chickpeas
- 1 medium size sweet potato cubed
- 1 teaspoon of cumin
- 1 teaspoon of curry powder
- 1 pinch of chili flakes
- ½ inch piece of ginger grated
- 1 tablespoon of chopped parsley

- 2 tablespoons flaxseed meal
- 1 tablespoon of organic tahini
- 1 tablespoon of tamari
- Sesame seeds to coat

Instructions:

Quick and Easy Sunflower Bread:
1. This is such a great recipe for raw bread! Simply place all of the ingredients in a bowl and mix very well to combine. Allow the mixture to stand for 15 minutes or so to absorb the water and then spread out on your teflex sheet around 1cm thick, covering the whole tray.

2. Dry at 105 degrees for 4 hours and then flip over and remove the teflex. Dry for another hour or two until the bread is dry through but still soft and malleable.

3. Cut each sheet into 9 even pieces and store in an airtight container in the fridge for up to 2 weeks.

Chickpea Burger Patties:
1. Place the chickpeas and sweet potato in your food processor and blitz until it is relatively smooth- a few chunks are ok! Add the remaining ingredients and process until everything is combined.

2. Roll into small patties in your hand and then flatten onto a dehydrator tray lined with a teflex sheet.

3. Scatter with sesame seeds and dehydrate for 6-8 hours at 105 degrees. Flip them over, remove the teflex and dehydrate until dry- another 2-4 hours. Store in an airtight container in the fridge for up to 2 weeks.

Assembly of Burger - The Whole Shebang:
1. If you are making the bread and patties, make those first. The raw versions will take at least 24 hours, the cooked patties will take an hour or so!

2. When you are ready and have your patties and bread on hand, prepare all of your salad ingredients and then simply stack the burger as you please. You can add a layering of lettuce, cucumber, tomato, carrot, hummus and onions.

Deviled NonEgg

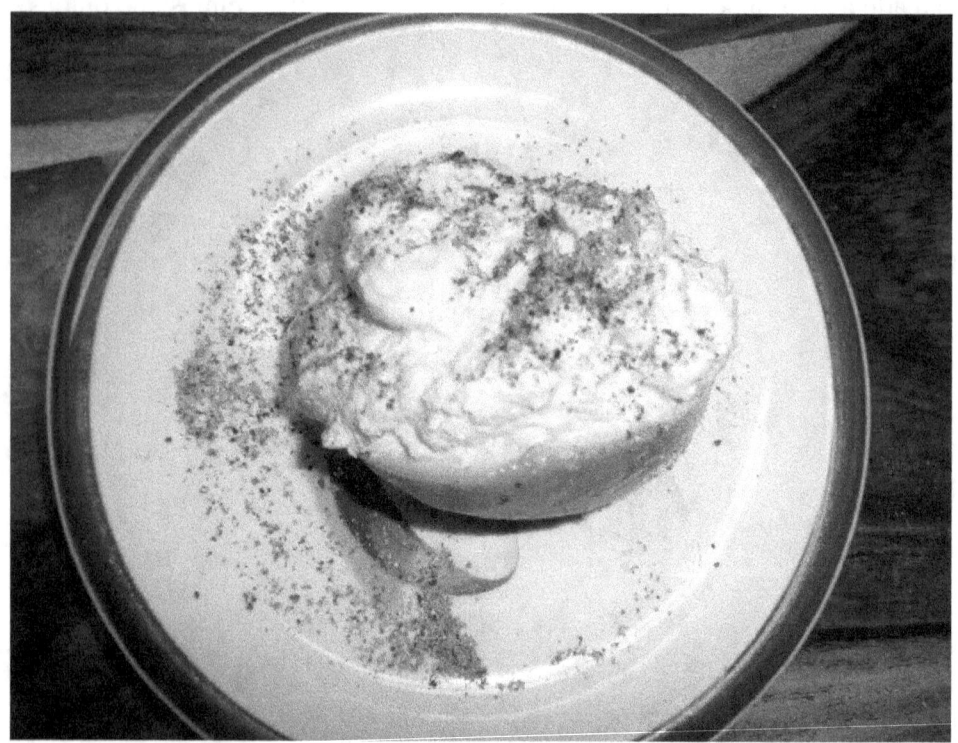

Ingredients:
½ cup raw mayonnaise (recipe is in this book)
½ cup fresh lemon juice
1 ½ teaspoons turmeric
2 cloves garlic, peeled
1 ½ teaspoons Himalayan black salt
1 ½ cups raw macadamia nuts (soaked)

Instructions:
We soak them over night but they can be soaked for a couple of hours. When ready, we then gather the following: ½ cup chopped onions ½ cup chopped celery 1/2 cup chopped red bell pepper.

In a high speed blender, combine the raw mayonnaise, lemon juice, garlic, salt and nuts and blend until smooth.

In a mixing bowl, combine the contents of the blender with the onions, celery and bell peppers. Mix well and serve. Top with black pepper.. enjoy!

Author's Note: To date, this is the best deviled egg raw, vegam recipe we have ever come across. Our staff at the clinic as well as our patinets absolutely rave about the realistic taste, in part because of the Himalayan Black salt. It can be found at many Asian food markets as well as on Amazon.

3.4 Desserts

Testing largely depends on the type of parasite. For example, pinworms are the most common parasites residing To test you will have to conduct a tape test for the diagnosis of Pinworm infection. This test is quite simple. All you have to do is to take a piece of cellophane tape and press its sticky side

Raw Coconut Carrot Cake

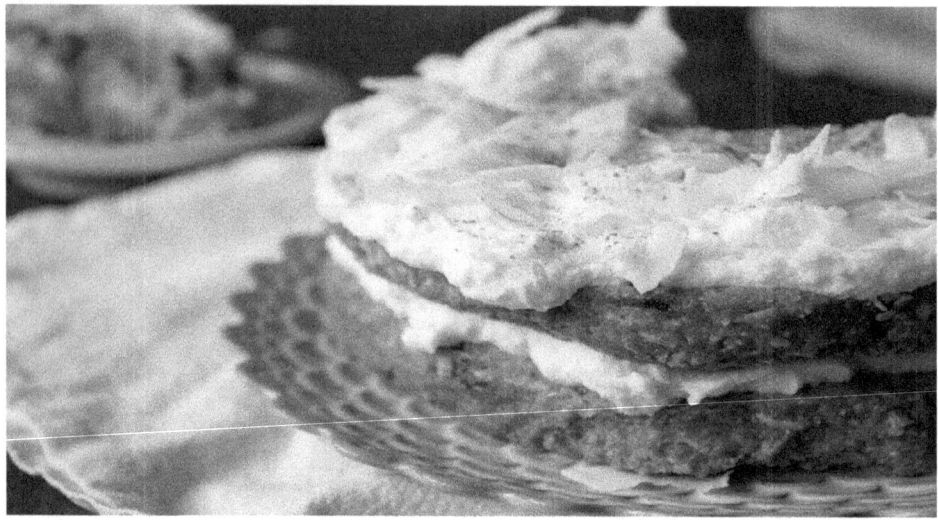

Ingredients:
- 1 cup pitted medjool dates
- 1/4 cup dried unsweetened pineapple, chopped
- 2 1/2 cups shredded coconut
- 1 cup walnuts
- 1 cup pecans
- 1 teaspoon fresh grated ginger
- 1 teaspoon cinnamon
- 1/4 teaspoon nutmeg
- 1/4 teaspoon allspice
- 1/8 teaspoon ground cloves

- dash of Himalayan pink crystal salt
- 1/4 cup coconut water
- 1 cup shredded carrot
- 1/4 cup raisins
- 1 cup coconut cream
- 1 tablespoon agave
- 3 tablespoons coconut flour

Instructions:

1. In a food processor combine fruit, 2 cups of coconut, nuts, and spices . Pulse until combined, but still a hearty crumbly texture.

2. Add the shredded carrot and coconut water, and pulse 5 times.

3. Remove the blade from the food processor, and add the raisins.

4. Use a wooden spoon to stir the ingredients together. The batter will be sticky, but it will firm up a bit in the fridge.

5. Draw a 5-inch diameter circle onto 2 separate sheets of parchment paper (you can trace a Pyrex bowl).

6. Place the parchment paper onto your counter, pencil/pen side down.

7. Scoot half of the carrot cake batter into the center of the circle, and smooth down with a spatula to make a cake layer. It should be about 1 inch thick.

8. Do this with the other circle and remaining batter.

9. Place the two halves into the fridge to firm for at least 30 minutes.

10. To make the icing combine the coconut cream, agave, and flour in a standing mixer and whip until fluffy and creamy. Or use a hand mixer to do this.

11. Place icing in the fridge to firm for at least 20 minutes.

12. Ice one of the cake layers with half of the icing.

13. Top with the other cake layer, and top with the remaining icing.

14. Garnish with remaining shredded coconut, a sprinkle of cinnamon, and serve!

Easy Peppermint Chocolate Fudge

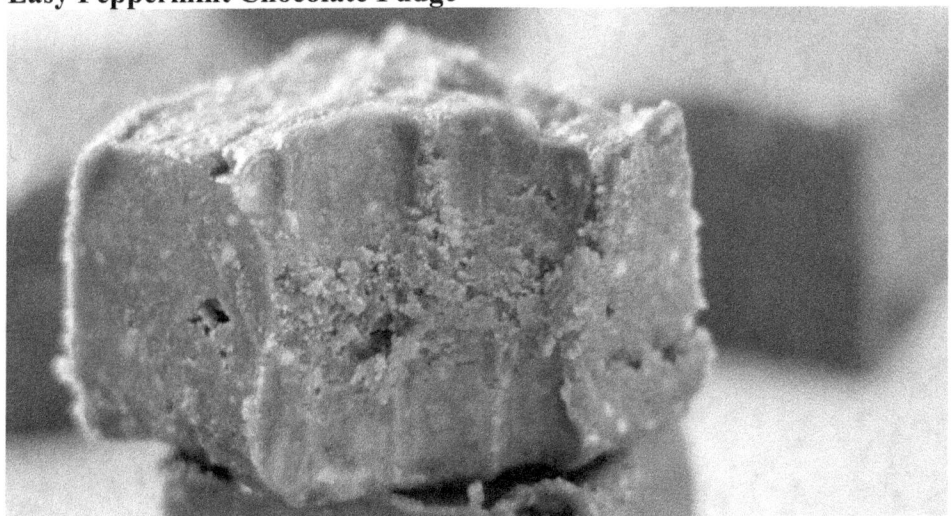

This easy peppermint chocolate fudge is made with only 5 ingredients and takes 5 minutes to make and 1 hour to set. It is infused with amazing peppermint essential oil.

Ingredients:
- 1 1/2 cashew butter
- 1/3 cup coconut oil, melted
- 1/3 cup raw cacao powder
- 2 tablespoons agave
- 6 drops peppermint essential oil

Instructions:
1. Add all ingredients to a blender/food processor and blend until smooth.

2. Spoon the mixture into a loaf tin lined with baking paper and smooth over with a spatula.

3. Place into the freezer for approximately 1 hour to set.

4. Take out of the freezer and cut into desired portion sizes.

Meyer Lemon Pie

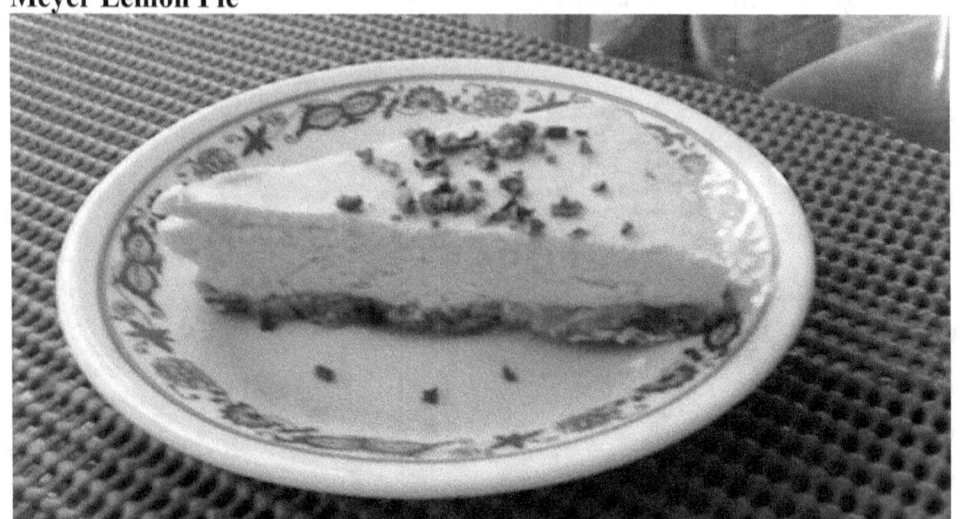

Ingredients:
Crust:
- 1 1/2 cups raw macadamia nuts
- 1 cup pitted dates
- 1/3 cup shredded coconut
- 2 tablespoons raw cacao nibs

Filling:
- 1 cup raw cashews
- 1 tablespoon coconut butter
- 6 Meyer lemons juiced
- 1 tablespoon coconut oil
- 1/2 teaspoon Himalayan pink crystal salt
- 1/4 to 1/2 cup organic raw agave
- 1/2 tablespoon vanilla extract (non-alcoholic, organic)

Instructions:
Crust:
1. Place all ingredients in a food processor or high speed blender. Process ingredients until well combined and sticky.

2. Press into the bottom of a slightly greased spring form, cheesecake pan, or Pyrex pie plate. Or, line with saran wrap.

3. Place in the freezer till ready to pour filling.

Filling:
1. Place all ingredients in a high speed blender. Mix on high until mixture is super smooth thick, and creamy. Taste filling, adjust sweetness as needed.

2. Pour filling over crust in pan. Smooth our filling. Cover with saran wrap and place in freezer.

3. Freeze for about 2 hours or more, until set. Garnish with raw cacao nibs, or sliced Meyer lemons.

Notes Store leftover pie covered in the freezer. Thaw slightly before serving.

Strawberry Vanilla Cashew Cake

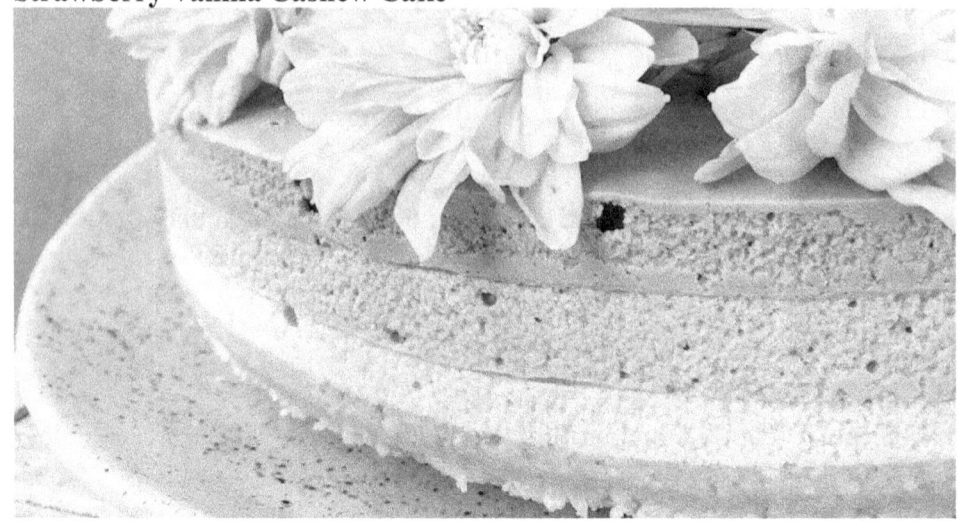

Ingredients:

Crust:
- 1 cup raw cashews
- 1 cup shredded coconut
- 1/3 cup rice malt syrup/agave/coconut nectar OR 10 pitted medjool dates
- pinch of sea salt

Vanilla "cheesecake" layer:
- 1.5 cup raw cashews (soaked)
- 1/3 cup melted coconut oil
- 1/3 cup light, liquid sweetener
- 2 tbsp lemon juice
- 1/2 tsp vanilla powder
- pinch of sea salt

Strawberry "cheesecake" layers:
- 3 cup raw cashews, soaked
- 2/3 cup melted coconut oil
- 2/3 cup light, liquid sweetener
- 2 tbsp lemon juice

- 1/2 tsp vanilla powder
- 1 cup fresh, or defrosted strawberries

For dark pink layer:
1-2 tsp beetroot powder

Instructions:
1. To make the crust, simply process cashews and coconut in a food processor until a fine flour. Add in your liquid sweetener of choice (or dates) and salt and process until everything sticks well together. Press the dough into a lined tin and set aside.

2. For the vanilla layer, blend all ingredients until completely smooth in a high speed blender. Spread over the crust and freeze until solid (1-2 hours or so).

3. For the pink layers, simply blend all ingredients (except beetroot powder) until smooth in the blender. Spread half of the batter over the vanilla layer and set away in the freezer to set. Blend the rest of the batter with the beetroot powder. Spread this on top of the cake. 4. Let the cake freeze for at least 2 more hours before serving. The cake can be served frozen, or you can let it defrost for a few hours on the kitchen table(or overnight in the fridge).

Decorate with fresh flowers or whatever else you have on hand.

Vegan Christmas Cheesecakes

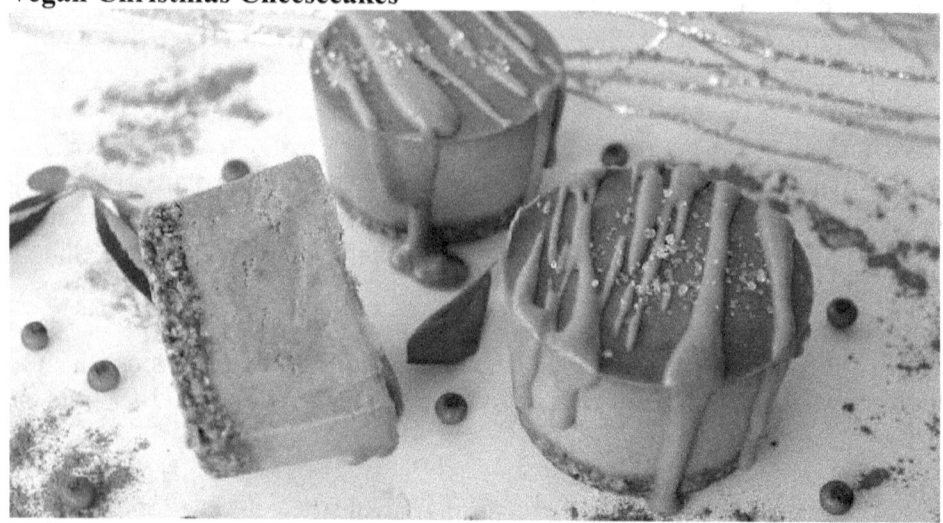

Ingredients:

Crust:
- 2/3 cup sunflower seeds or almonds
- 2/3 cup shredded coconut
- 1 cup raisins
- 1 teaspoon water

Filling:
- 2 cups raw cashews
- 1 cup water
- 5 tablespoons coconut nectar
- 1 teaspoon pure vanilla extract
- 1/2 cup melted coconut oil
- 4 tablespoons melted coconut butter
- 1 1/2 - 2 tablespoons whole greens powder
- Beet root powder, for desired color

Drizzle:
- 2 cups • 2 tablespoons hot water, or more
- 2 tablespoons melted coconut butter

- 1 1/2 tablespoons melted coconut oil
- Beet root powder, as desired pieces

Instructions:

Crust:
1. Grind the seeds and coconut in a food processor.
2. Add the raisins and process until they're combined.
3. Add the water and pulse a few times. The mixture should easily stay together when pressed in your hand.
4. Press into the bottom of pan(s) of choice.

Filling:
1. Blend the cashews, water, nectar, and vanilla until smooth in a high speed blender.

2. Add the oil and butter. Blend again to incorporate.

3. Pour 1/3 of the filling into a bowl and stir in some beet powder.

4. Add the green powder to the remaining 2/3 of the filling in the blender and blend. Pour the green filling over the crusts, leaving some space at the top.

5. Add a big spoonful of beet filling on top and use the spoon to push it down into the green filling. Spoon a little green filling over the top.

6. Chill in the freezer for at least 6 hours, remove the silicone molds or spring form pan and place in the fridge for at least 6 hours.

Drizzle:
1. Whisk all ingredients together until smooth. If it's too thick to drizzle, add a touch more water. Just a little to start so that it doesn't get runny. It will firm up quickly on the cold cakes.

Raw Caramel Apple Pie

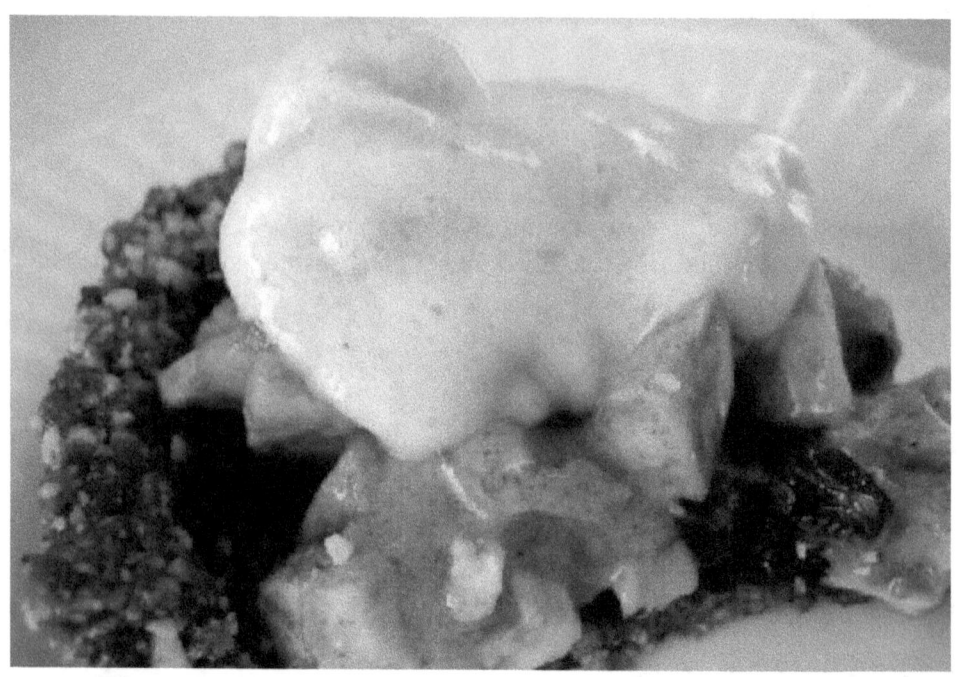

Preparation Time: 20-30
Servings: 6
"Cooking" Time: 120

Ingredients:
Filling:
5 apples, peeled and sliced
1/8-inch thick
1/2 cup raisins
4 tablespoons agave
4 tablespoons lemon juice
1 teaspoon cinnamon
1/2 teaspoon pumpkin pie spice

Crust: 1 cup walnuts
1 cup raisins

Caramel: 4 tablespoons almond butter
2 tablespoons agave
2 tablespoons olive oil
4 tablespoons water

Directions:
1. For filling, in a lidded container (I used a zip lock box), toss the apples and 1/2 cup raisins with the agave, lemon juice, cinnamon, and pumpkin pie spice until well coated. Spread out on a lined dehydrator sheet and dry for about 2 hours, stirring once or twice. This isn't meant to dry the apples, but to soften them and let the flavor intensify.

2. For crust, in a food processor fitted with the "S" blade, process the walnuts and 1 cup raisins until the mix starts to stick together. This takes a couple minutes. Press the mix into the bottom and 2 inches up the sides of an 8 inch spring form pan. Put in the freezer for a half hour to firm.

3. For the caramel, in a bullet type blender, puree the almond butter, agave, olive oil, and water until very smooth. Spoon the apple mixture from the dehydrator into the chilled pie crust and pour the caramel evenly on top. Chill for another half hour, if desired.

Raw Choco Chip cookies

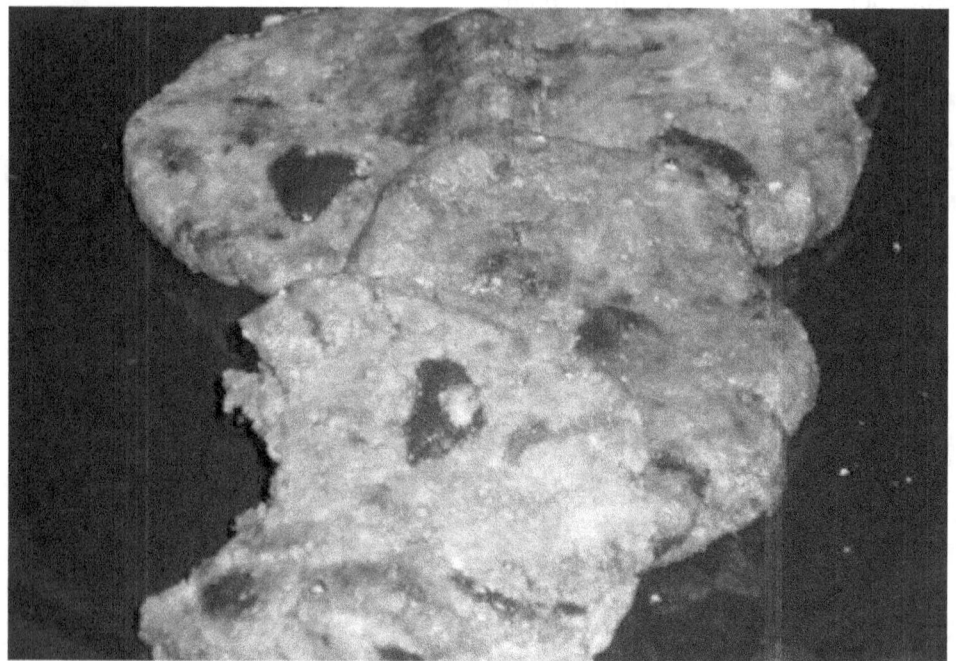

Preparation Time: 20 minutes
Servings: 4
"Cooking" Time: 15 minutes

Ingredients:
Dough: 1 cup cashew flour (grind raw cashews in coffee grinder)
1/2 cup whole oat groats (grind in coffee grinder)
2 tablespoons agave nectar
2-3 tablespoons coconut oil

Coco chunks:
1/2 cup or more of vegan cocoa/carob chips (optional)

What I do though:
1/4 cup coconut oil melted
4 tablespoons cacao powder
1-2 tablespoons of agave (depends on preference for sweetness).

Directions:

Mix the chocolate chips mix together and freeze in a pan. Do it quickly to avoid the coconut oil getting hard again. When you take it out after about 15 minutes (depending on thickness), break into tiny chunks. Mix all of the dough ingredients together. (Use your hands, it's easiest).

Now fold in the chocolate chip chunks. Form into cookie shapes and place in dehydrator for 15- 20 minutes to get warm and hold shape. OR you can put in the refrigerator and eat them cold. Be sure to store these in the fridge though.

Raw Chocolate Cake

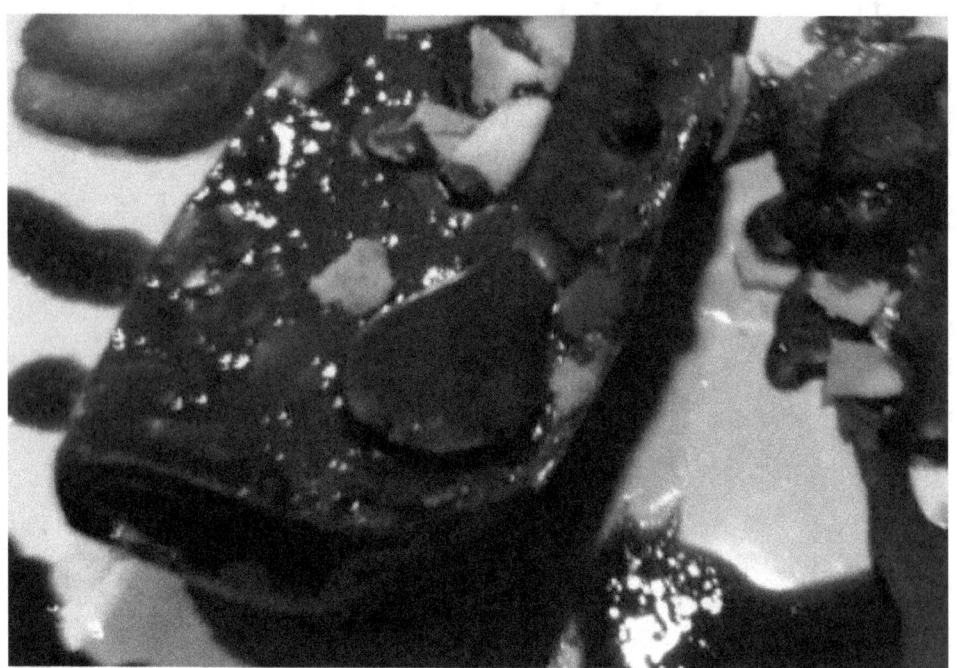

Preparation Time: 30-60 minutes

Ingredients:
Crust: 3/4 cup almonds, soaked for 30 minutes if you have time
1/2 cup dried coconut
1/3 cup coconut oil, melted
1-2 tablespoons almond or peanut butter
1-2 tablespoon cacao powder water, as needed

Filling:
1 avocado sweetener, to taste (I use coconut sugar, agave syrup, dates, or apple juice)
3-4 tablespoons cocoa or cacao powder
vanilla essence or fresh orange juice, to taste
3/4 cup soaked irish moss, and blended well with water Chocolate sauce, optional: 1/4 cup coconut oil, melted cacao powder, to taste

Directions:
1. For crust, grind together the first 5 crust ingredients until you get a crumbly base type mixture. I did it in the Vita-mix. Add water if needed, and press into a cake tin.

2. For filling, in a powrful blender, mix the filling ingredients together until you get a super-thick chocolaty moussey-type consistency. I blended this in the Vita-Mix.

3. Decorate with coconut and fruit of your choice. The irish moss gives it a special jelly type texture, enabling you to cut the cake. For chocolate sauce, mix chocolate sauce ingredients, and drizzle over top, if desired. If you don't have irish moss, add 1-2 avocados and 1/2-1 cup soaked cashew nuts into the mix and blend on high until thick. Pour on to base, and put in refrigerator or freezer to set. Sweeten to taste.

Raw Chocolate-Mint Pie

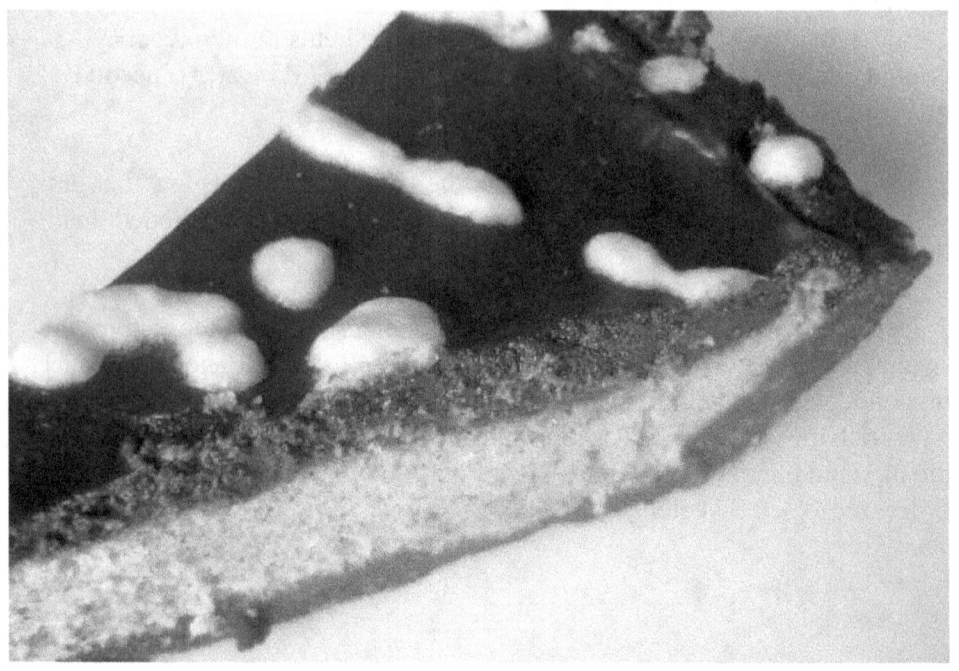

Preparation Time: 20 to 30 minutes
Servings: 1

Ingredients:
Crust:
3/4 cup almond flour
1/2 cup packed dates
1/2 cup pecans
1/4 cup cacao powder
2 tablespoons coconut oil
1/2 teaspoon vanilla extract
pinch salt.

Filling:
2 large avocados
1/2 cup melted coconut oil

1/4 cup agave syrup
2 teaspoons mint extract, or to taste
1 tablespoon fresh or dried mint leaves
1 teaspoon lemon juice

Ganache:
1/2 cup cacao powder
1/4 cup agave syrup
2 tablespoons water
2 tablespoons coconut oil
pinch salt

Drizzle:
1/4 cup soaked cashews
2 tablespoon agave syrup
1/4 teaspoon vanilla extract
1 tablespoon coconut oil
Water, to thin

Directions:
1. Crust: In the bowl of a food processor, place all crust ingredients; process until well combined. Press into an 8-inch pie plate or tart pan. Chill until firm.

2. Filling: In the clean bowl of a food processor, place all filling ingredients; process until well combined and creamy. Pour filling into crust; chill until set.

3. Ganache: In another bowl, place all ganache ingredients; combine until smooth. Pour ganache over filling in a thin layer. Chill until set.

4. Drizzle: In the clean bowl of a food processor, place all drizzle ingredients; process until well combined. Drizzle over top or pipe through a piping bag.

5. Freeze for a more ice creamy pie or chill for a softer pie.

RAW Dark Chocolate Brownie Balls

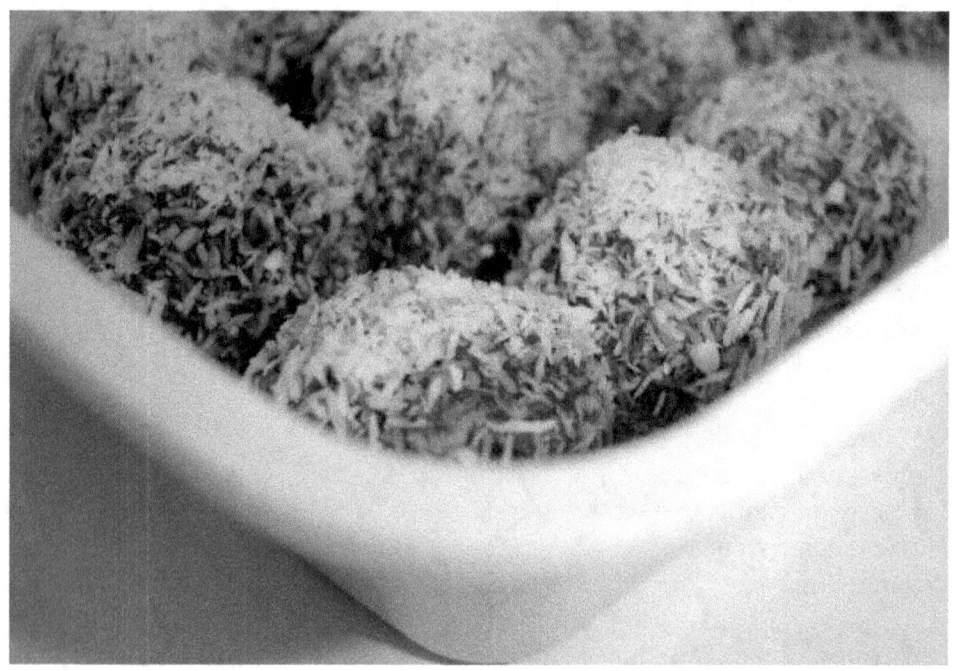

Preparation Time: 15 to 20 minutes
Servings: 6 to 12

Ingredients:
1 cup raw sunflower seeds, soaked then sprouted for 1 day
1/4 cup raw cacao powder
3 tablespoons raw mesquite powder
3 tablespoons raw agave nectar or 5 to 6 halawi dates, pitted
1 cup raw shredded unsweetened coconut.

Directions:
1. In a food processor, grind the sunflower seeds to a gritty pulp. Stir in cacao and mesquite, process again.

2. Stir in dates or agave, process again until the dough clumps together and collects at one side of the food processor.

3. Transfer the dough to a bowl, and shape into approximately 1" diameter balls. Roll balls into the coconut and refrigerate until ready to serve. These will keep for 2 days in the fridge, when you preroll the balls. Add coconut shreds before serving. The dough can be frozen, but thaw out approximately 30 to 45 minutes prior to rolling in the coconut and serving.

Variations: Substitute raw hemp seeds for shredded coconut, for an alternate taste with a nice added crunch. Substitute raw Mesquite for raw Maca, for an alternate taste, but still just as tasty.

Giovanna's RAW Tiramisu

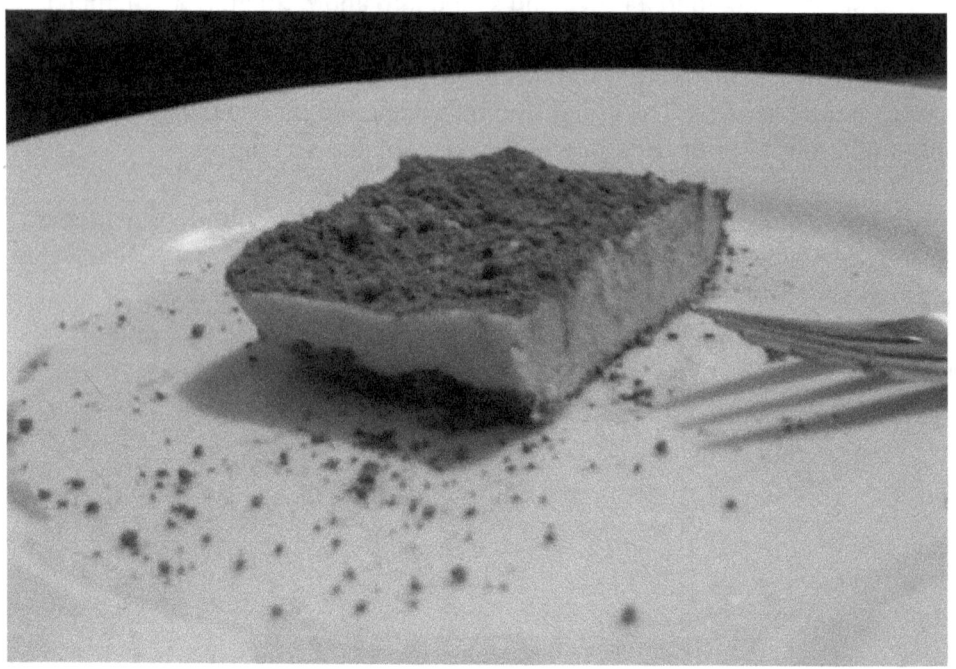

Preparation Time: 1 hour
Servings: 2-4
"Cooking" Time: 1 hour

Ingredients:
2 cups macadamia nuts, soaked 4-6 hours
1/2 cup cashews, soaked 4-6 hours
2 tablespoons agave nectar
1/4 teaspoon almond extract (or part of a vanilla bean)

Crust:
1 cup dates, soaked 1 hour
3/4 cup ground pecans
1/4 cup ground flax seed cocoa powder or finely cut cacao chips

To serve:

4 tablespoons maca 'coffee', prepared

Directions:
1) In a food processor or blender, blend together the macadamias and cashews, scraping often if necessary. Be sure to get it ultra creamy. Add agave and almond extract and blend to mix. Pour into a bowl and set aside.

2) Process the dates by themselves until very mushy. Add in the pecans and flax and blend until a dough forms.

3) Press the dough into a small pan or make individual servings by pressing into a cupcake pan. Make sure the dough is even and not too thick.

4) Scrape the nut filling mixture onto the crust and gently smooth. Sprinkle cocoa on top and refrigerate for at least one hour.

5) Pour a tad of the 'coffee' onto you plate and serve the piece on top. Enjoy! Will keep a few days in fridge or a month in freezer. This freezes and thaws very well.

Raw Ice Cream Sandwiches: Two Ways

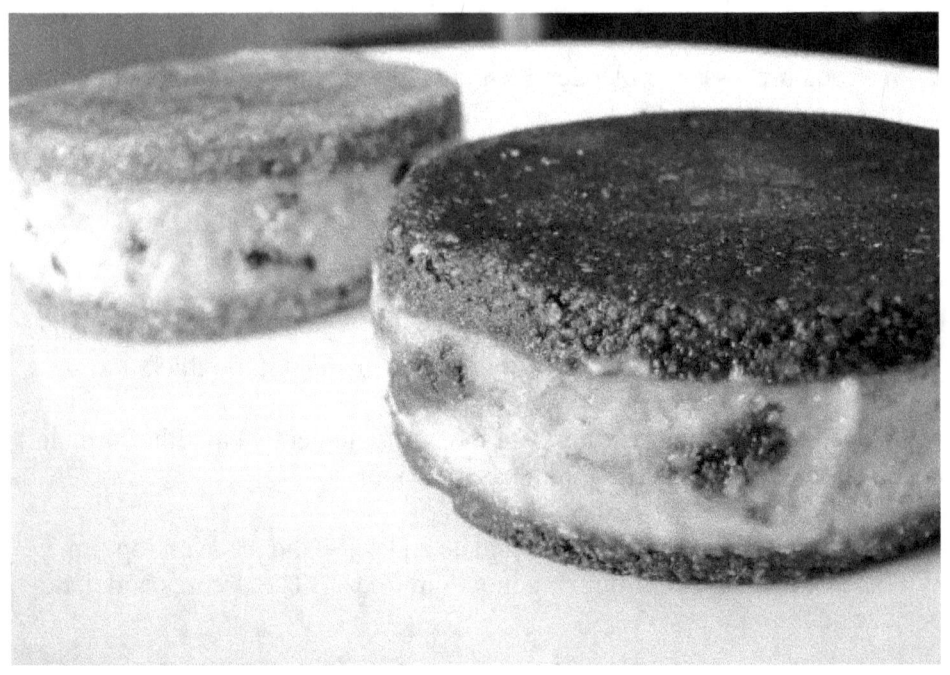

Preparation Time: 30 minutes
Servings: 4
"Cooking" Time: 5-6 hours

Ingredients:
Ice Cream:
2 cups almond milk (1 cup almonds to 1 1/2 cups water)
1/2 cup hemp seeds
6 soaked medjool dates
1 tablespoon coconut oil
1 teaspoon vanilla pinch salt

Oreo (Chocolate) Cookie:
1/2 cup almond flour
1/2 cup unsweetened shredded coconut, ground fine
1/4 cup raw cacao powder

1/4 cup agave/or other syrup sweetener
2 teaspoons mesquite powder
pinch salt
1 tablespoon coconut oil

Chocolate Chip Cookie:
3/4 cup almond flour
1/2 cup unsweetened shredded coconut, ground fine
1/4 cup agave
1 tablespoon mesquite powder
pinch salt
2 tablespoons cacao nibs.

Directions:
1. Combine almond milk, hemp seeds and dates in a blender. Blend until uniformly smooth. Drain mixture through a sieve to strain out any date/hemp clumps. Return mixture to blender, and add add coconut oil, vanilla and salt. Blend until combined. Make ice cream according to ice cream maker instructions.

2. Assemble ingredients for chocolate/oreo cookies (except coconut oil) in a medium bowl. Roll with a rolling pin until 1/4" thick. Cut four 4" circles out of it, put on dehydrator tray and dehydrate at 115 degrees F for 6 hours or until firm-ish.

3. With the leftover dough, add 1 tablespoon coconut oil, knead together, and form into flat shapes. Put shapes in freezer until firm (a few minutes). Spoon half of the ice cream into a bowl, chop the freezer dough into pieces and crumble into ice cream. Stir until combined.

4. Assemble ingredients for chocolate chip cookies in a medium bowl (except cacao nibs). Roll with a rolling pin until 1/4" thick. Cut six 4" circles out of it, put on dehydrator tray and dehydrate at 115 degrees F for 6 hours or until firm-ish.

5. You may have leftover dough, so if that is the case you could possibly get away with making a few extra (7-8). Spoon the other half of the ice cream into a bowl; add cacao nibs. Stir until combined. Once cookies are

dehydrated, spoon appropriate ice cream mixture onto cookie (the ice cream should be really smooth and malleable, perfect just out of the ice cream maker) top with another cookie, smooth sides with a knife. Freeze until firm.

Lemon Creme Pie with Carob Nut Crust

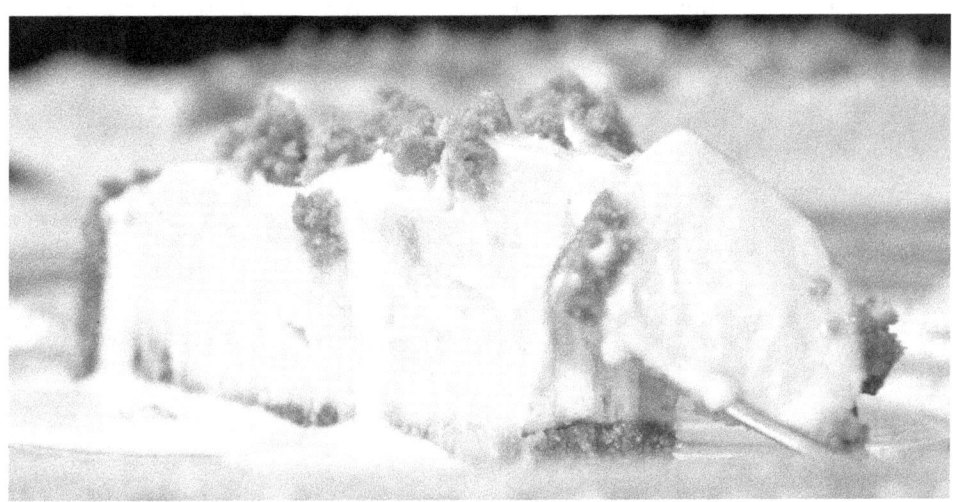

Preparation Time: 15 minutes
Servings: 2-6

Ingredients:
handful of raw cashews
handful of raw almonds
handful of organic dates
2 tablespoons carob powder
1 banana
1/2 cup shredded (unsweetened) coconut
2 tablespoon freshly squeezed lemon juice
1 tablespoon flaxseed oil

Directions:
Put cashews, almonds, dates and carob powder in processor to combine into breadcrumb-like texture. Add just enough water so that mixture combines.

Press mixture into pie plate lined with saran wrap (cling film). Put in freezer to set for about 5 minutes Rinse processor. Add to processor banana, coconut, lemon juice and flax oil and blend till creamy and smooth.

To serve: Lift up crust, peel of saran wrap and put back on plate. Spread lemon creme on base. Serve.

Raw "Maple"-Cinnamon Coconut Cookies

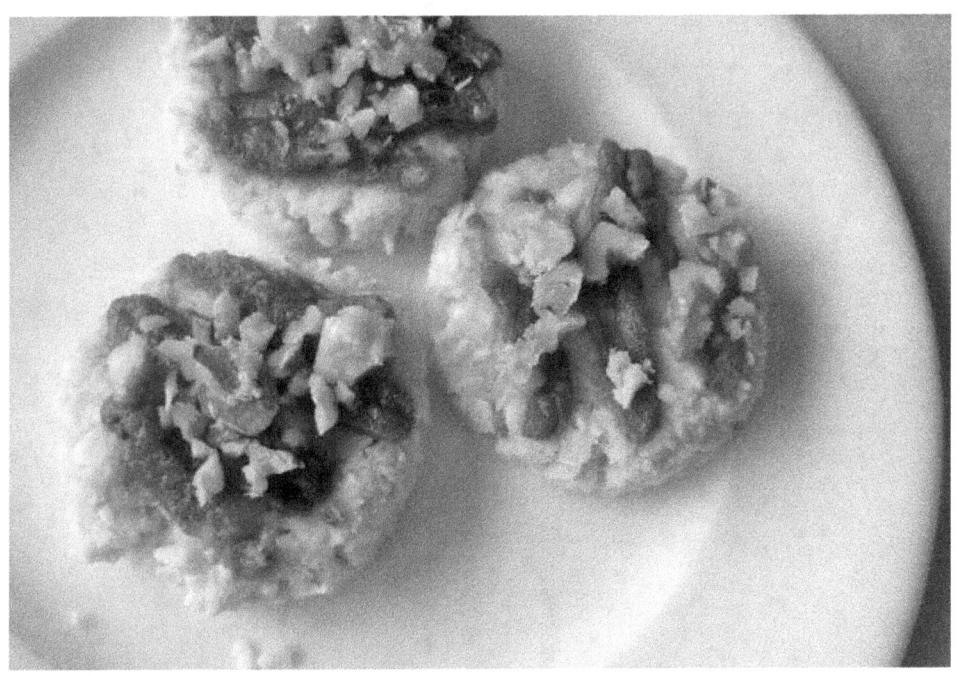

Preparation Time: 10 minutes
Cooking time: 0 min
Servings: 20

Ingredients:
Cookies:
2 cups shredded coconut
6 tablespoons coconut flour
1/4 cup + 2 tablespoons agave
1 teaspoon vanilla extract or ground vanilla beans
4 tablespoons melted coconut oil

"Maple" Cinnamon Icing:
1/4 cup packed dates
2 tablespoons agave syrup
1/2 teaspoon cinnamon

2 teaspoons coconut oil
water to thin, as needed nuts, to taste, for topping.

Directions:
1. Combine all ingredients for cookies. Roll into balls.

2. Place on a wax paper lined flat surface and press into a round cookie shape.

3. Combine ingredients for glaze in a food processor. Pipe onto cookies. Top with nuts. Freeze until hardened.

Peaches N Cream Pie

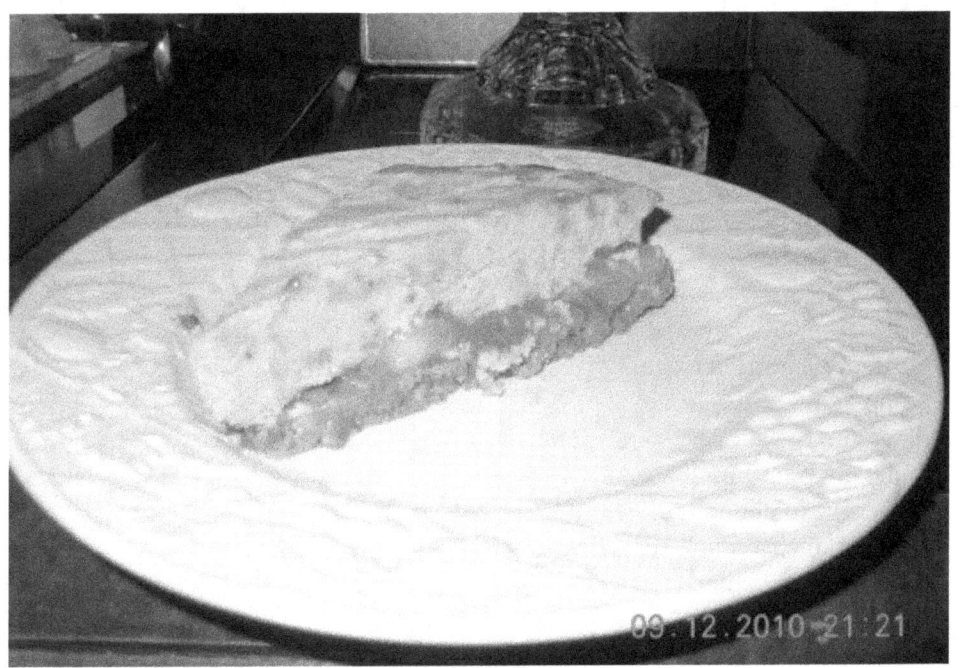

Preparation Time: 1 day
Servings: 1

Ingredients:
Crust: 1 1/4 cups raw pecans, chopped finely
1/3 cup oat flour (process raw oat groats in food processor into flour; sift)
1/8 teaspoon sea salt
4 dates
1 tablespoon virgin coconut oil, plus more for pan

Peach Filling:
2 yellow peaches
Skinned and chopped 5 white peaches, skinned and chopped
3 teaspoons cinnamon
1/4 teaspoon nutmeg
1/4 teaspoon cloves

1/2 teaspoon arrowroot
3/4 cup agave nectar
5 dates
1/2 teaspoon vanilla extract
1 1/2 teaspoons molasses
pinch sea salt

Cream Topping:
1 cup raw cashews
1 vanilla bean
1 tablespoon cocoa butter
1 tablespoon vanilla extract
1/2 cup agave
3 dates
1/4 cup coconut butter
1/2 cup virgin coconut oil
1/8 teaspoon + a pinch sea salt
1/4 teaspoon all spice.

Directions:
1. For crust, combine oat flour, pecans and salt, then set aside. Process dates and coconut oil until a thick paste is formed. Combine all ingredients with hands. Mix well. Grease the bottom of a 10 1/2 inch pie pan with about a dime size amount of coconut oil. Cover the bottom and side of the pie pan with crust mixture. Dehydrate at 110 degrees for at least 45 minutes.

2. For filling, place all peaches in bowl, and add cinnamon, nutmeg, cloves, sea salt and arrowroot. Set aside. Process "maple" Syrup, agave nectar, dates, vanilla, and molasses in the food processor until smooth. Add mixture to peaches. Mix well then fill the pie crust with mixture. Dehydrate at 110 degrees for 4-6 hours.

3. For topping, soak cashews and 1/2 vanilla bean in water for 2-6 hours. Drain cashews and vanilla bean, and then place in the food processer. Process for 30 seconds, add 1 tablespoon of water and process for another 30 seconds, repeat once more. Heat cocoa butter on low until melted, then remove from heat and set aside.

4. Combine all ingredients except cocoa butter in food processer, process until smooth. Add cocoa butter and process until smooth. Put mixture over the peach pie and cover with plastic wrap. Place in the freezer for 1 1/2 hours. Refrigerate over night. Store in the fridge.

Raw Brownies!

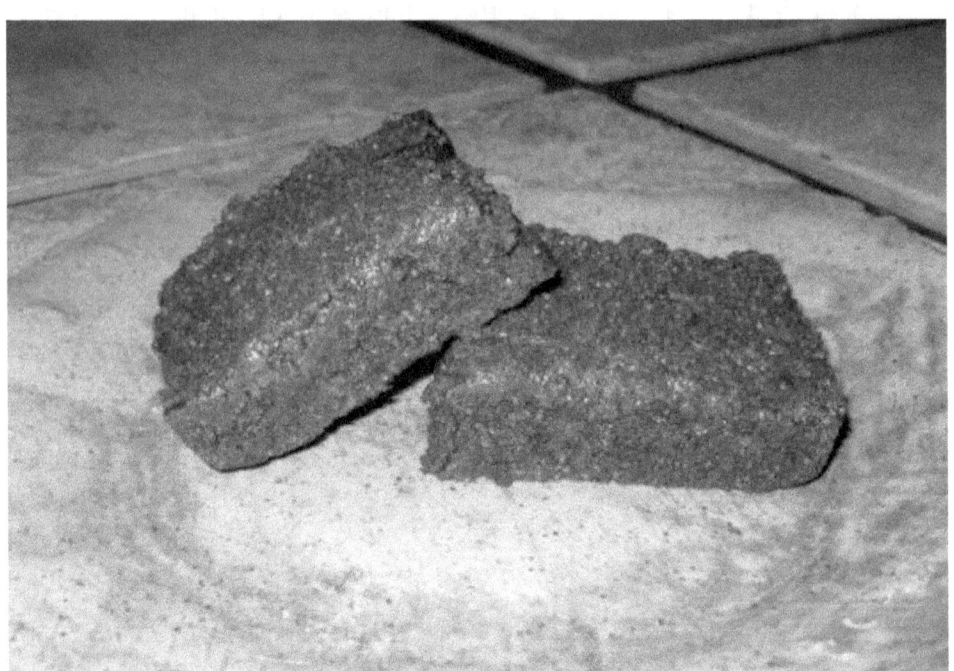

Preparation Time: 20 minutes
Servings: 2 to 4

Ingredients:
1 cup ground pecans
1 cup dates (not soaked)
1/4 heaping cup cocao powder
1 heaping teaspoon agave nectar

Icing:
1 tablespoon coconut oil or coconut butter
1 tablespoon avocado (optional)
1 tablespoon agave
1/2 tablespoon cocao powder.

Directions:

1) Process the brownie ingredients. Press into a pan or bowl.

2) Now process icing ingredients. If you use the coconut oil right out of the jar (firm) it should get very creamy in your food processor. If you do it by hand, warm up the oil jar in a bowl of water and use it in liquid form.

3) Spread frosting onto brownies and refrigerate for at least ten minutes. Slice and enjoy!

Raw vanilla ice cream with raw chocolate.

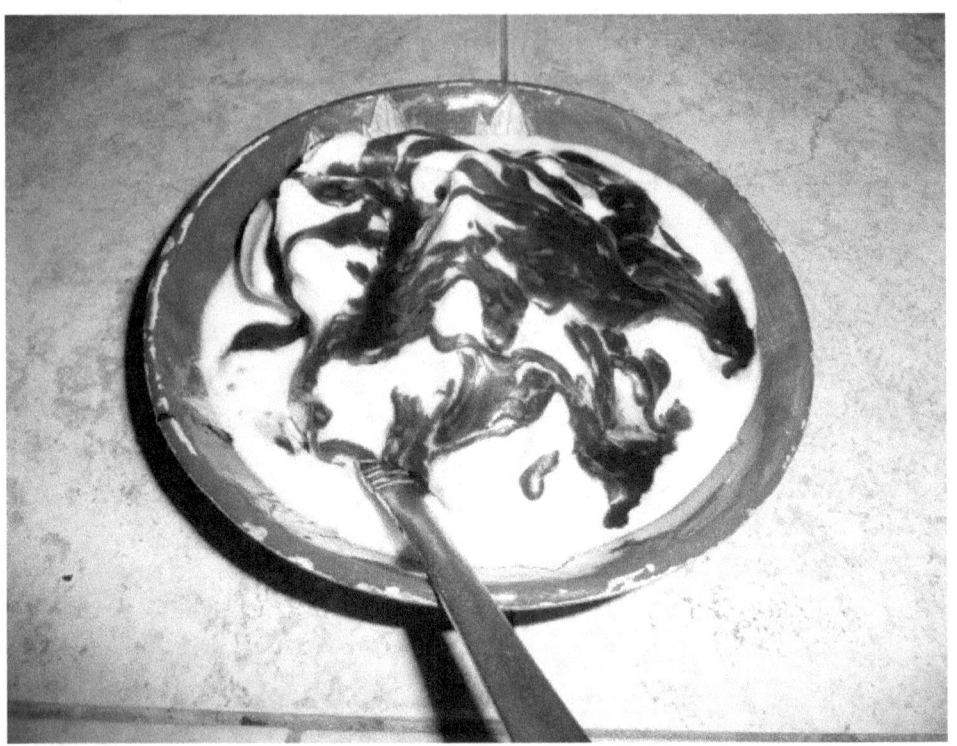

Ice cream:
1/4 cup Cashews
1 tablespoon vanilla
3 tablespoons agave (more if you like it sweeter)
2 cups ice. Blend till smooth.

Chocolate syrup:
2 tbsp coconut oil
2 tbsp raw cacao powder(we buy ours off Amazon)
1 tbsp agava
1/4 tsp vanilla mix with a fork.

Pour the syrup over the ice cream and eat it up! ***TIP*** You do NOT soak the cashews. Just put them in the blender and add your Vanilla and

Agave with about 2 tablespoons of water and blend till smooth. This is the trick to having it smooth. Then you add your ice and blend till smooth.

Apple Cinnamon "Toast"

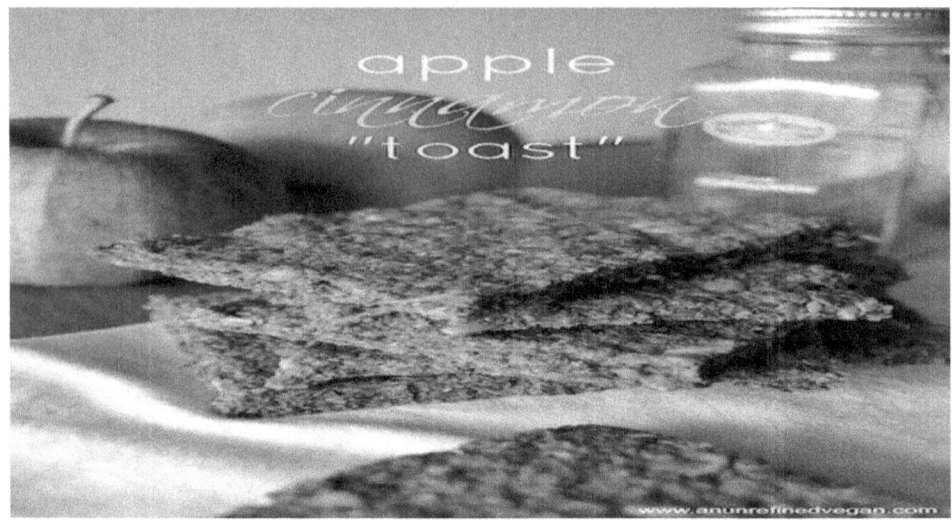

Ingredients
- 1 cup walnuts, soaked overnight
- 5 dates, soaked for about 15 minutes • 1 apple, cored
- 1 small sweet potato, peeled and cut into small pieces (about 1 cup)
- 1/2 cup unsweetened apple juice
- 1/2 of a banana
- 1 1/2 teaspoon cinnamon
- 1/4 teaspoon cardamom
- Pinch of Himalayan pink crystal salt • 1 cup flaxseed meal
- 1/4 cup flaxseeds
- 1/4 cup Raw Organic Hulled Sesame Seeds
- 1/4 cup raw hulled hemp seeds

Instructions:
1. In a food processor, process the walnuts through the salt until nearly smooth. You'll need to scrape down the bowl of the processor a few times.

2. In a large bowl, combine the flaxseed meal, flaxseeds, sunflower seeds, and hemp seeds.

3. Spread the mixture onto a dehydrator sheet to just a hair under 1/2" thick and neaten up the edges.

4. Gently score the dough into desired shapes. 5. Place in the dehydrator and dehydrate 105-degrees F for 60 minutes, then turn down the temperature to 105-degrees F and continue to dehydrate the "toast" until it is dry and very crispy, about 20-24 hours.

Raw cheesecake recipe

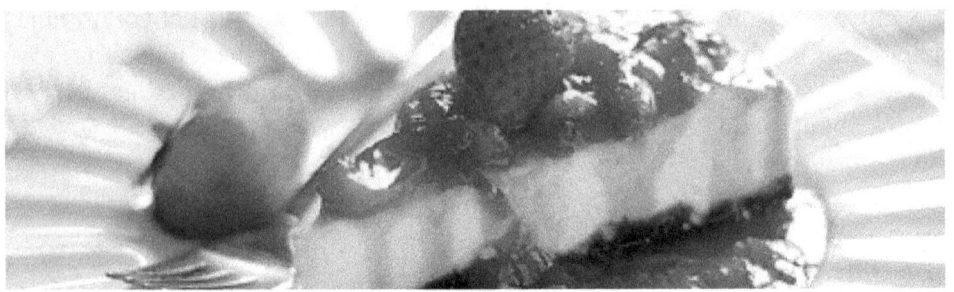

1 1/2 cups macadamia nuts (or a combination of walnuts and macadamia nuts)
1/2 cup dates
1/4 cup dried, unsweetened coconut
1 pinch sea salt

White cheesecake filling ingredients:
3 cups cashews
3/4 cup lemon juice
3/4 cup agave
3/4 cup coconut oil
1 tablespoon vanilla
Up to a 1/4 cup of water, if necessary to facilitate blending

Fruit topping ingredients:
2 cups frozen strawberries
1/2 cup dates

Preparation Time: 15 min
Wait Time
    2 hours

Total Time
    2 hours 15 min

Serving Size
    10 servings

Shelf Life
    1 week in freezer

Equipment
    Blender Food Processor

Directions:
How to make this raw cheesecake recipe...

1. Throw the macadamia nuts, salt and dates into your food processor. (Don't add the coconut!!) Process nuts and dates until well processed but still airy.

2. Next, get our your cheesecake pan (or just a basic glass brownie pan if you're like me and don't have fancy cookware) and sprinkle the coconut on the bottom as your very first layer. The point of doing this is to make it so it's easier to remove the cheesecake and the coconut stops the crust from sticking to the bottom of the pan. Then press the macadamia nuts and date mixture down into the pan to form the crust.

3. Throw all cream-cheese filling ingredients into your high-speed blender and blend! Add as little water as necessary to facilitate blending. (Try to add as little water as possible.) Pour mixture on top of crust.

4. Place the above in freezer for an hour or so (so that it will firm up).

5. Meanwhile, throw your strawberries and dates in your high-speed blender. Blend until nice and smooth. Pour this mixture on top of the crust/cream cheese, which was just in the freezer for about an hour. Place the raw cheesecake recipe back in freezer. Freeze until this raw cheesecake recipe reaches the desired consistency (5 hours or so!).

6. Defrost this raw cheesecake recipe for about a half-hour before eating (or just slice from freezer and enjoy this delicious raw cheesecake)!

The Rawtarian's Thoughts

This is an awesome raw cheesecake recipe. Will you believe me when I say that it tastes exactly like standard American diet (SAD) cheesecake? No, of course you won't believe me that this raw cheesecake recipe tastes just like the real thing. But it does!!

This is a three-stage process, which is a little more complicated than I normally work. But, it is important to have some kind of fancy dessert in your arsenal to impress the non-raw people in your life. This raw cheesecake recipe does the trick, hands down!

Plus, it's actually not that hard to make. Seriously.
This raw cheesecake recipe just takes three easy steps: crust (easy, throw in food processor and press down into pan); "cream cheese" (easy, throw everything in high-speed blender and pour on top of crust); and sauce (easy, throw everything in high-speed blender and pour on top). Enjoy this raw cheesecake recipe!

This raw cheesecake recipe is very rich, so it can serve, like, 20 people or something crazy like that!

Raw rice pudding

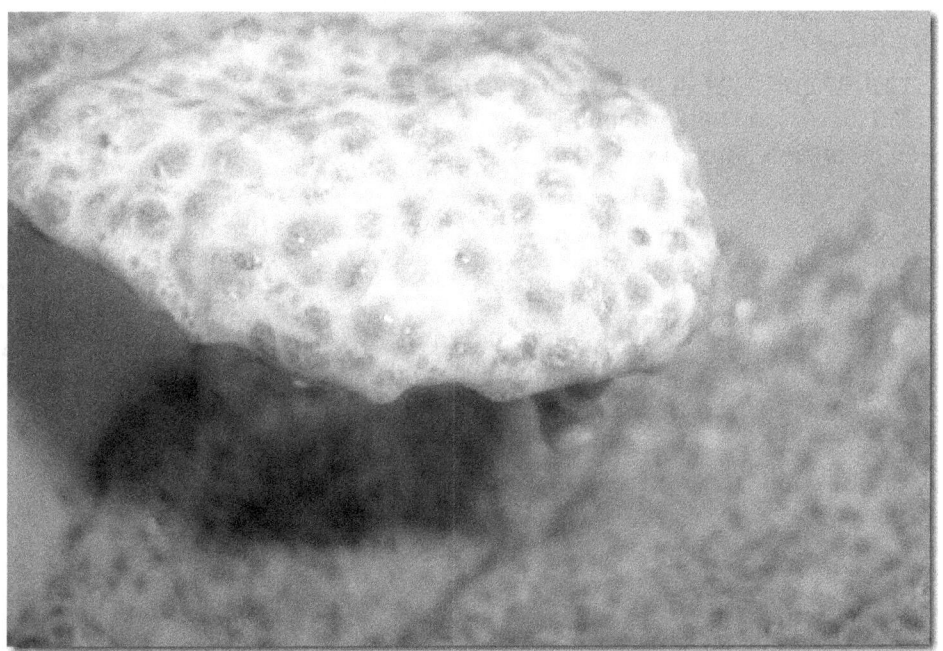

Ingredients
1 cup cashews
2 cups water
2 tablespoons agave nectar
1 tablespoon vanilla
1 tiny splash almond extract
1 teaspoon cinnamon
Small pinch sea salt
1/4 cup chia seeds (reserve)
1/4 cup raisins (reserve)

Preparation Time: 5 min
Wait Time: 3 hours
Total Time: 3 hours 5 min
Serving Size: 3 servings
Shelf Life: 3 days in fridge

Equipment: Blender

Directions:
Directions re: how to make raw rice pudding
1. Put all ingredients (except the chia seeds and the raisins) in a high-speed blender and blend until smooth.

2. Place chia seeds and raisins in a large bowl. Pour the blended mixture on top of the chia seeds and rasins, mixing slowly and thoroughly.

3. Cover raw rice pudding mixture and refrigerate for at least one hour. The purpose of refrigerating and letting the mixture sit for at least an hour is to allow the chia seeds to absorb the liquid. (Chia seeds are similar to tapioca. They increase in size!) Ideally, let this recipe sit in fridge for 3 hours. Overnight is even better!

4. Stir thoroughly before serving.

Raw food eggnog recipe

Ingredients
5 ripe bananas
1 cup cold water
1 tablespoon agave nectar
1 tablespoon coconut oil or coconut butter
2 teaspoons vanilla extract
1/2 teaspoon cinnamon
1/8 teaspoon cloves
1/8 teaspoon allspice
1 pinch of sea salt

Preparation Time 5 min

Serving Size 1 large smoothie
Shelf Life Consume immediately
Equipment Blender

Directions
1. Blend until smooth.

2. Taste. Add more cinnamon, cloves or allspice to taste.

3. Consume immediately. If refrigerated, the texture will change and become more of a pudding, so consume this raw food eggnog recipe immediately.

3.5 Snacks

Apricot Chia Energy Bars

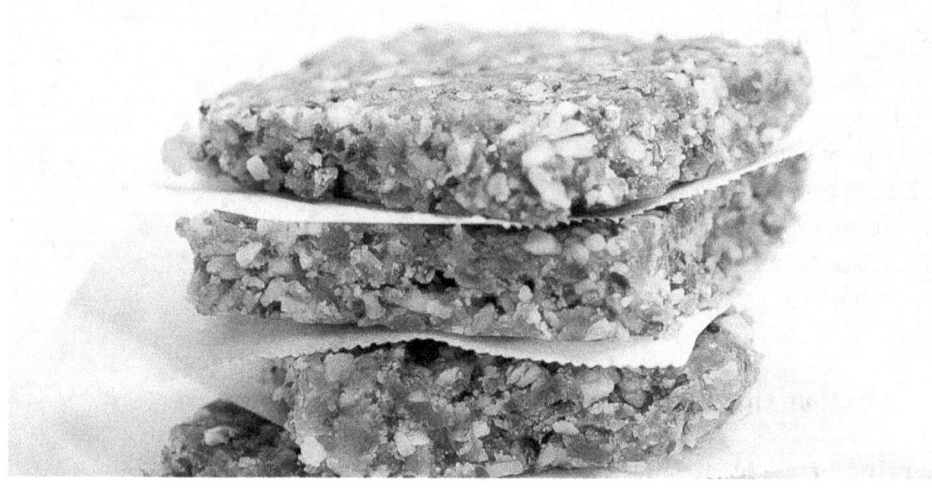

Ingredients:
- 1 cup dried apricots
- 1 cup pitted dates
- 2 tbsp chia seeds
- ¼ tsp cinnamon
- ½ cup raw pumpkin seeds
- ½ cup hemp seeds
- 2 tbsp coconut oil melted

Instructions:
1. Line a 8x8 or 9x9 square pan paper.

2. Place dates, apricots and cinnamon in a blender, and pulse several times until dates and apricots turn into chunks.

3. Add pumpkin, chia seeds and coconut oil to the mixture in the blender, and pulse until there are small chunks of pumpkin seeds

4. Press the mixture into the prepared pan. Roll the top with a glass to flatten completely.

5. Refrigerate for 45 minutes.

6. Slice into bars or squares.

Banana Pops

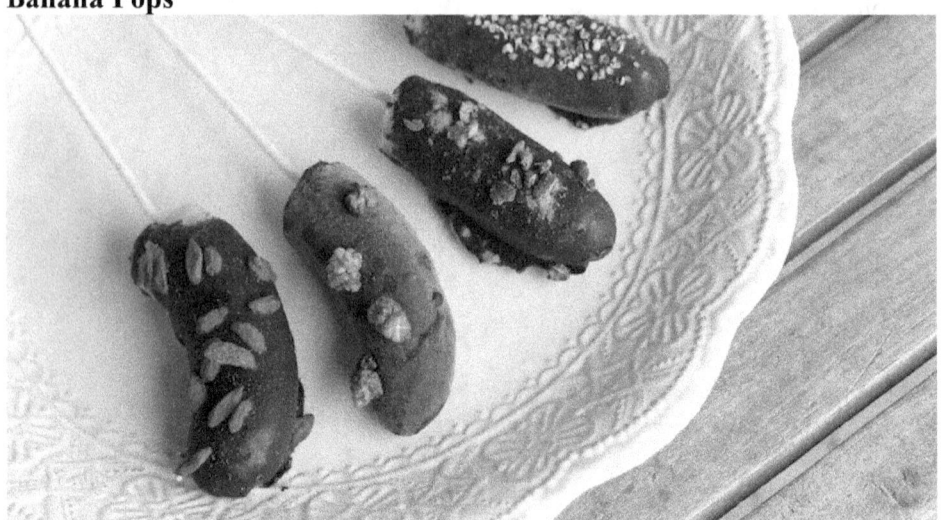

Ingredients:
- 3 Bananas, halved & frozen
- ⅓ cup Coconut Oil
- ⅓ cup cacao powder
- 3 tbsp Organic agave Syrup
- Superfoods to top

Instructions:
1. Peel and cut your bananas in half. Carefully add a stick and freeze on parchment for a few hours or overnight.

2. In a small mug or bowl, melt your coconut oil and mix in the cacao powder till fully combined. Mix in your agave

3. The next step takes some quick hands, you want to dip and coat each banana pop as quickly and evenly as possibly - while coating them before the mixture hardens into a shell. So setting out your toppings ahead of time is vital for them to stick properly.

4. Cover with your favorite superfoods, you can go crazy with combos!

Cheeze Crackers with Peanut Butter

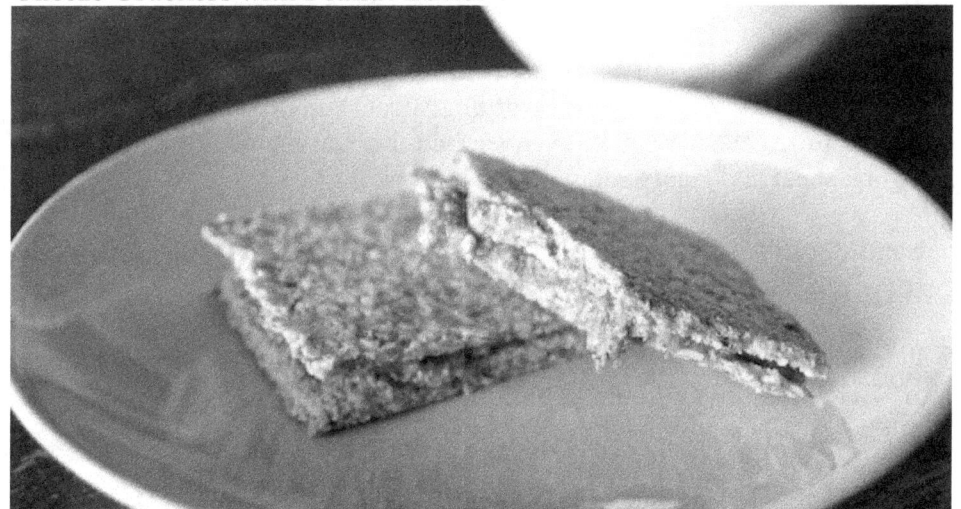

Ingredients:
- 1 cup flaxseed meal
- 1/4 cup raw coconut flour
- 1/2 cup nutritional yeast
- 2 medium-sized carrots, peeled and cut into chunks
- 1 apple, cored and cut into chunks
- 1 1/2 cups Almonds, soaked for 8-10 hours, rinsed and drained
- 1/4 cup coconut oil, melted
- 1 cup water • 1 tsp. white miso
- 1 Tbsp. agave syrup

Instructions:
1. In a large bowl, combine the flaxseed meal, coconut flour and the nutritional yeast. Set aside.

2. In a food processor, grind the almonds into a crumbly meal - don't over process, otherwise you'll have almond butter. Not a bad thing, but not what you're looking for here. Empty the almond meal into the bowl w/ the flaxseed mixture. Process the carrots and apple until you have a nice mash. Scrape the mixture into the big bowl.

3. Add the remaining ingredients and stir until thoroughly mixed. The mixture should be moist but hold together when pressed.

4. Divide the mixture in two and spread one half on a dehydrator tray that has been covered with a non-stick drying sheet. You'll just about be able to cover the full sheet. To get an even surface, I cover the dough with another non-stick sheet and gently roll with a rolling pin.

5. Carefully lift off the non-stick sheet. Once the dough has been rolled out, gently score the surface into squares.

6. Place the trays in the middle of the dehydrator and set the temperature to 115F. Dehydrate for 68 hours or until the cracker are very crispy all the way through.

7. About halfway through the process, I carefully transfer the dough to a dehydrator screen.

Raw Coconut Carrot Cake

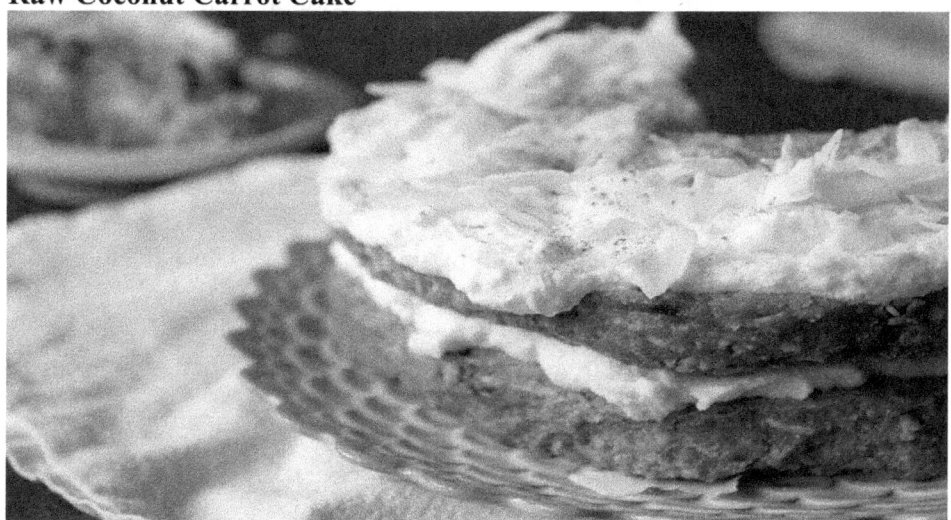

Ingredients:
- 1 cup pitted medjool dates
- 1/4 cup dried unsweetened pineapple, chopped
- 2 1/2 cups shredded coconut
- 1 cup walnuts
- 1 cup pecans
- 1 teaspoon fresh grated ginger
- 1 teaspoon cinnamon
- 1/4 teaspoon nutmeg
- 1/4 teaspoon allspice
- 1/8 teaspoon ground cloves
- dash of Himalayan pink crystal salt
- 1/4 cup coconut water
- 1 cup shredded carrot
- 1/4 cup raisins
- 1 cup coconut cream
- 1 tablespoon agave
- 3 tablespoons coconut flour

Instructions:
1. In a food processor combine fruit,

2 cups of coconut, nuts, and spices . Pulse until combined, but still a hearty crumbly texture.

2. Add the shredded carrot and coconut water, and pulse 5 times.

3. Remove the blade from the food processor, and add the raisins.

4. Use a wooden spoon to stir the ingredients together. The batter will be sticky, but it will firm up a bit in the fridge.

5. Draw a 5-inch diameter circle onto 2 separate sheets of parchment paper (you can trace a Pyrex bowl).

6. Place the parchment paper onto your counter, pencil/pen side down.

7. Scoot half of the carrot cake batter into the center of the circle, and smooth down with a spatula to make a cake layer. It should be about 1 inch thick.

8. Do this with the other circle and remaining batter.

9. Place the two halves into the fridge to firm for at least 30 minutes.

10. To make the icing combine the coconut cream, agave, and flour in a standing mixer and whip until fluffy and creamy. Or use a hand mixer to do this.

11. Place icing in the fridge to firm for at least 20 minutes.

12. Ice one of the cake layers with half of the icing.

13. Top with the other cake layer, and top with the remaining icing.

14. Garnish with remaining shredded coconut, a sprinkle of cinnamon, and serve!

Cookies with Strawberry Jam

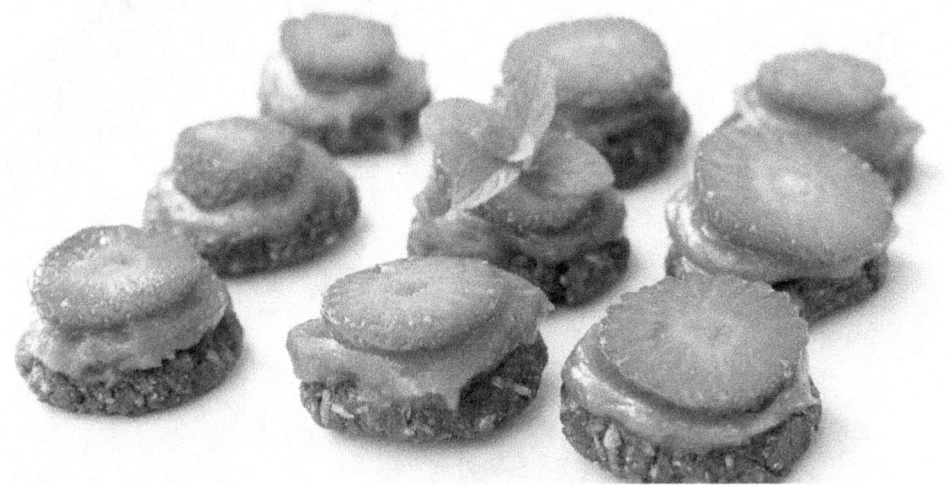

Ingredients:
Cookies:
- 2 cups dates
- ⅓ cup shredded coconut
- 2 Tbsp carob flour
- 1 tsp vanilla powder

Strawberry Jam:
- 2 cup fresh strawberries (or thawed frozen)
- 2 cups dates

Decoration:
- ¼ tsp vanilla powder
- Fresh strawberries

Instructions:
1. In a food processor mix dates, add coconut flakes, carob and vanilla and mix until it sticks together.

2. Form cookies.

3. For the strawberry jam, mix everything in a blender until smooth.

4. Put a little bit of jam on each cookie and decorate with a slice of strawberry. Enjoy!

Easter Macaroon Nests

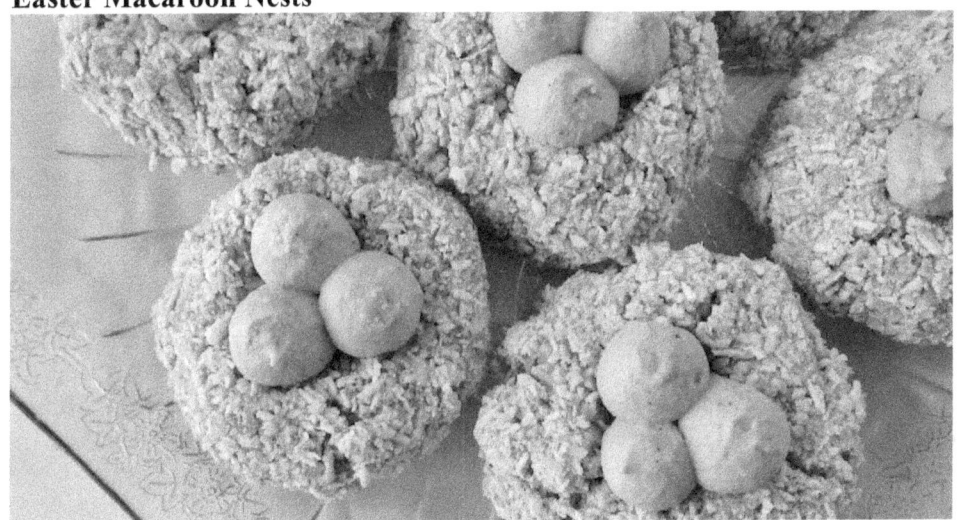

Ingredients:
Macaroons:
- 3/4 cup raw almond meal*
- 2 Tbsp organic lime zest
- 2 Tbsp lime juice
- a pinch of sea salt
- 1/4 cup raw coconut nectar
- a few spinach leaves
- 2 cups finely shredded coconut

Cream "eggs":
- 1/2 cup raw cashews (preferably soaked overnight)
- 2 Tbsp lime juice
- 1 /2 Tbsp organic lime zest
- 1/2 cup fresh young coconut meat (or additional soaked cashews if not available)
- 2 Tbsp raw coconut nectar
- 1/8 tsp sea salt
- 1 teaspoon pure vanilla extract
- 2 Tbsp coconut butter, warmed to soft
- 2 Tbsp raw coconut oil (warmed to liquid)

- 1/4 cup fresh organic strawberries

Instructions:

1. Place almond meal, lime zest, lime juice, and sea salt in the food processor and process until well combined.

2. Add the agave nectar and spinach and process until the mixture holds together.

3. Add coconut and pulse until the mixture holds together.

4. Form the mixture into 12 balls, then press down in the center of each to form a nest and place on a dehydrator sheet. Dehydrate for about 12 hours, or until they are dried, but not so much so that they are not a little chewy in the middle.

5. To make cream, combine all ingredients except coconut oil and berries in the food processor and process until smooth.

6. With the motor running, add the oil slowly and process a minute.

7. Add the berries and process until well blended.

8. Place in a bowl in the freezer to firm up for about 30 minutes.

9. Place the cream in a pastry bag with a large round tip (or a ziplock with the end cut off) and pipe eggs into the nests. Enjoy! Store extra in the fridge.
Notes

*I used soaked, skinned and dried almonds to make the meal.

Mini Lemon Coconut Cookies

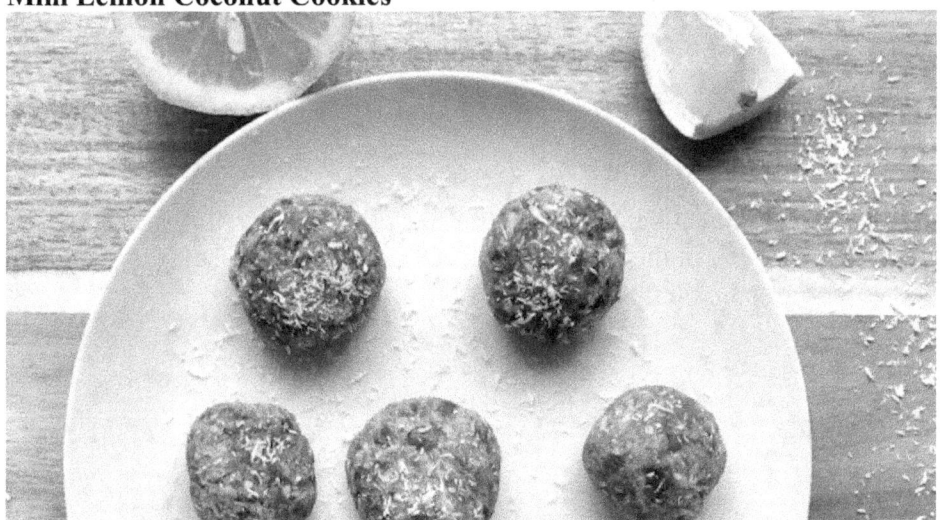

Ingredients:
• 10 pitted Medjool dates (if yours aren't pitted, remove the pits before making this recipe)
• 1/3 cup shredded coconut (finely shredded)
• juice from 1/4 a lemon (about 1 tbsp. of lemon juice)

Instructions:
1. First, you'll need to soak the dates to soften them up. Put them in a bowl and cover them in cold water and them put them in the fridge overnight. Or you can soak them in a bowl covered in warm water for one hour and leave them out on the counter if you forget to soak them overnight in the fridge. When you're ready to make the recipe, drain the dates and discard the soaking water. Put them on a paper towel and pat dry just enough to remove any excess water dripping from them.

2. Put the dates in the food processor or a mini food chopper (just put them in whole), or you can put them in the short cup of a Nutribullet .

3. Add the coconut into the machine on top of the dates and then add the lemon juice. Puree/blend until you get a thick cookie dough and that's when you know you're done!

4. Next, scoop out the dough with a spoon and roll into small balls about the size of a quarter each.

5. Put each cookie on a glass plate to set, or you can put them in a glass reusable storage dish.

6. Add any additional shredded coconut if you want a pretty garnish. Store these for one week in the fridge or you can freeze them in baggies and keep in the freezer up to a month.

Oat Free Hazelnut Cacao Truffles

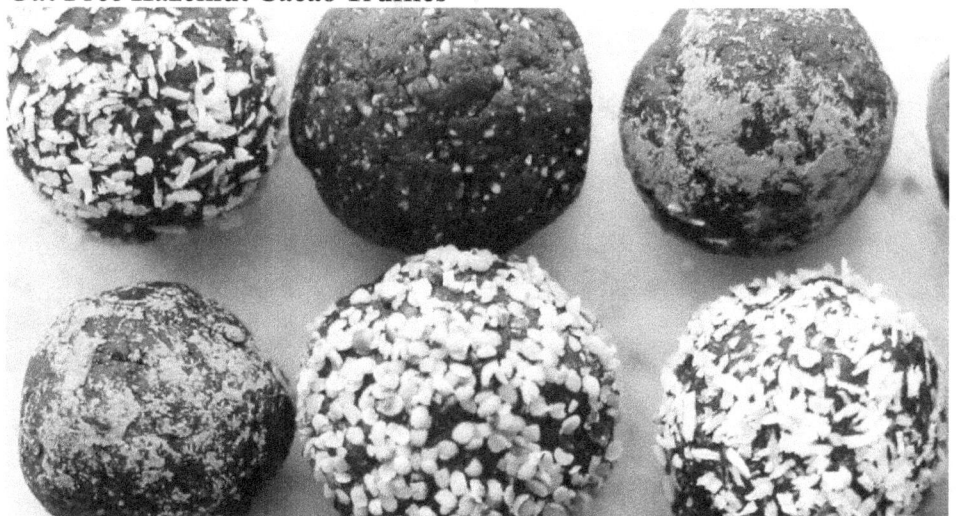

Ingredients:
- 1 cup raw hazelnuts
- 1 cup cashews
- ¾ cup cacao powder
- ½ cup coconut flour
- 3 tablespoons raw hemp seeds
- ¾ cup filtered water
- 15 medjool dates, pitted
- 2 tablespoons cacao nibs

Instructions:
1. In a food processor, process hazelnuts, cashews, cacao powder, coconut, and hemp till a flour like consistency.

2. Add water and dates, then continue blending till ingredients form a dough.

3. Pulse in cacao nibs, then remove dough from food processor.

4. Divide dough into 18 even pieces, using your hands, roll each piece into a ball.

Notes Refrigerate in airtight container up to one week, or in freeze up to one month.

Pizza Crackers With Avocado Dip

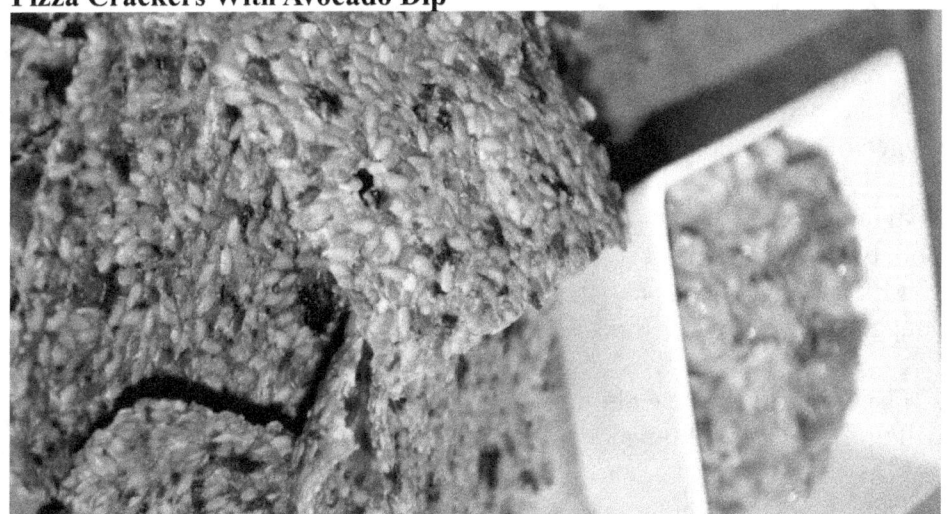

Ingredients:
Dough for crackers:
- 1/2 cup of grounded flaxseed and 1 1/2 cup flaxseeds soaked in approx. 2 cups of water for about 4 hours
- 1/4 cup sunflower seeds, grounded
- 2 tablespoons of dried majoram or a cup of fresh majoram
- 5 cloves garlic
- 2 teaspoons salt (depends on your taste)

Dough for pizza crackers:
- 1/2 cup of grounded flaxseed and 1 1/2 cup flaxseeds soaked in approx. 2 cups of water for about 4 hours
- 1/4 cup sunflower seeds, grounded
- 1/4 cup pumpkin seeds, grounded
- 1/4 cup dried tomatoes, soaked until soft
- 1/2 chopped onion
- 1 teaspoon olive oil
- 2 clove garlic, crushed
- 1 teaspoon tamari
- 1 tablespoon of spices of your choice
- 1/3 cup of raw olives, chopped

- generous pinch of black pepper add salt if needed Avocado dip
- 1 ripe avocado
- 1 clove garlic
- 1/2 red bell pepper
- 2-3 cherry tomatoes
- pinch of salt and black pepper

Instructions:
Both types of crackers:
1. Mix all ingredients together in food processor until you get a sticky dough. Add more water if needed.

2. Place your dough evenly on non-sticky sheets (about 1-2cm thick). You will probably use 2-3 trays.

3. Dehydrate for 6 hours at 115 degrees, then cut in squares, remove the sheets and dehydrate for another 6 hours.

Avocado Dip:
1. Blend all ingredients in food processor and serve with crackers.

Simple Savory Crackers

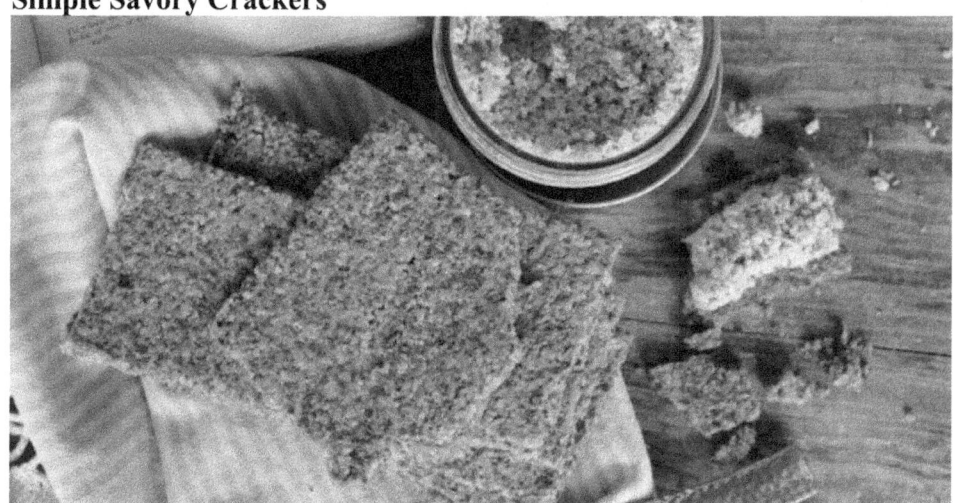

Ingredients:
- 2 cups walnuts
- 1 cup hemp seeds
- 1 cup grated carrots
- 1 tablespoon of fresh herbs (rosemary, thyme, sage)
- 1 tablespoon shallot, minced
- 2 tablespoons extra virgin olive oil
- 1/4 cup water (more if needed, should be a firmer constancy, but easily spreads onto dehydrator sheets)
- 1/4 cup flaxseeds, ground

Instructions:
1. In a food processor, grid the walnuts and then add hemp seeds, carrots, herbs, shallot, oil and water.

2. Process until you reach your desired texture.

3. Pour into a bowl and add in ground flax.

4. Let firm up then spread on to the teflex sheets, cut into desired size.

5. Dehydrate at 115 degree for 10 hours or until crispy!

Walnut and Mint Stuffed Dates

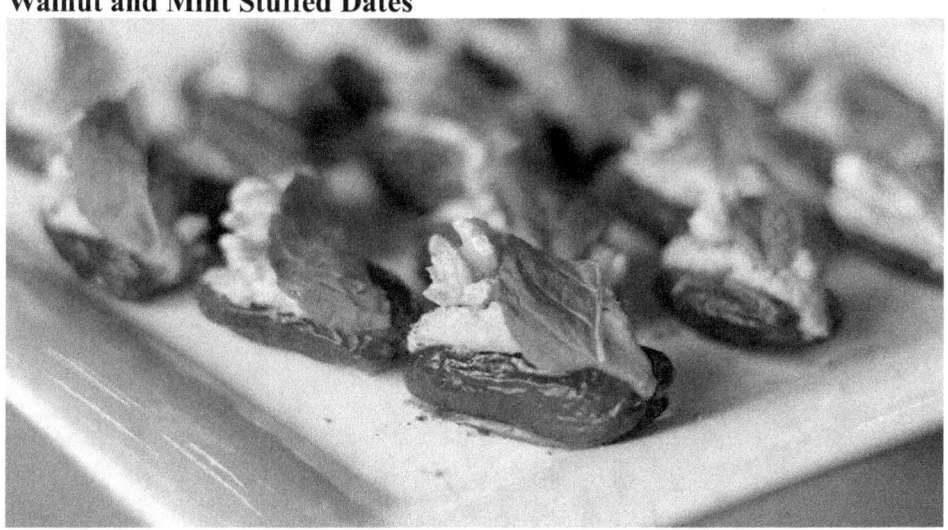

Ingredients:
- 20-30 dates (amount will vary based on size of dates)
- 1/2 cup raw cashews, soaked for 30+ minutes, drained & rinsed
- 1/2 cup raw walnuts, soaked 30+ minutes, drained & rinsed
- 1 tablespoon lemon juice
- Zest of 1 lemon
- 1/4 teaspoon Himalayan pink crystal salt
- 1 tablespoon agave
- 1 tablespoon olive oil
- 20-30 walnut halves, for garnish
- 20-30 mint leaves, for garnish

Instructions:
1. In a high-speed blender, combine the cashews, walnuts, lemon zest and juice, sea salt, agave, and olive oil. Blend until smooth.

2. Remove all pits from dates and slice in half. Fill each date with a teaspoon or so of the nut mixture. Top with a walnut half and a mint leaf.

Watermelon Strawberry Pops

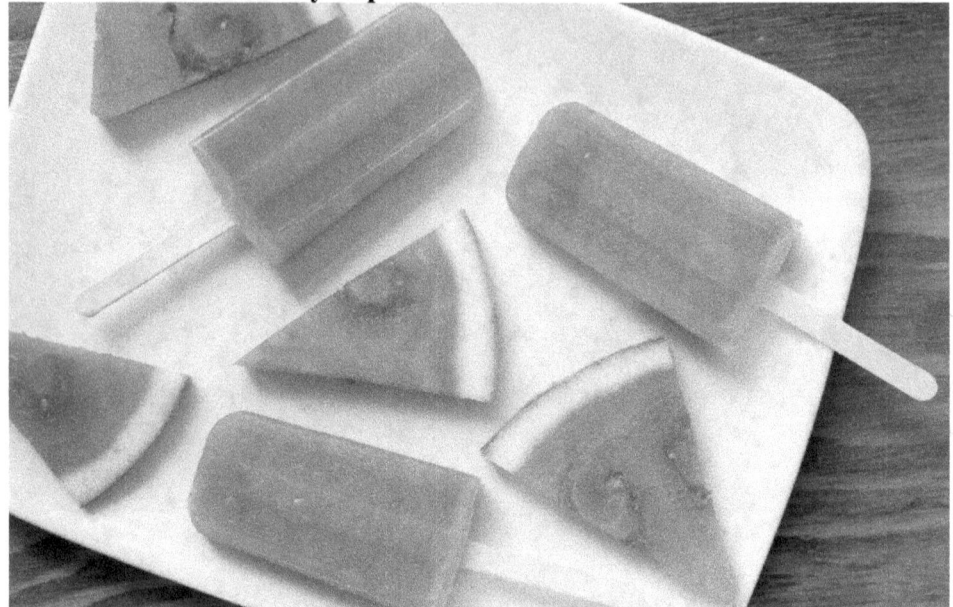

Ingredients:
- 2 cups watermelon chunks
- 1 cup strawberries
- 2 teaspoons agave
- Juice of 1/2 lemon

Instructions:
1. Using a high speed blender, puree the watermelon, strawberries, and the lemon juice together. Sweeten, if desired. Pour into popsicle molds and insert sticks,

2. Freeze for a couple hours, and enjoy!!

Raw corn chip recipe

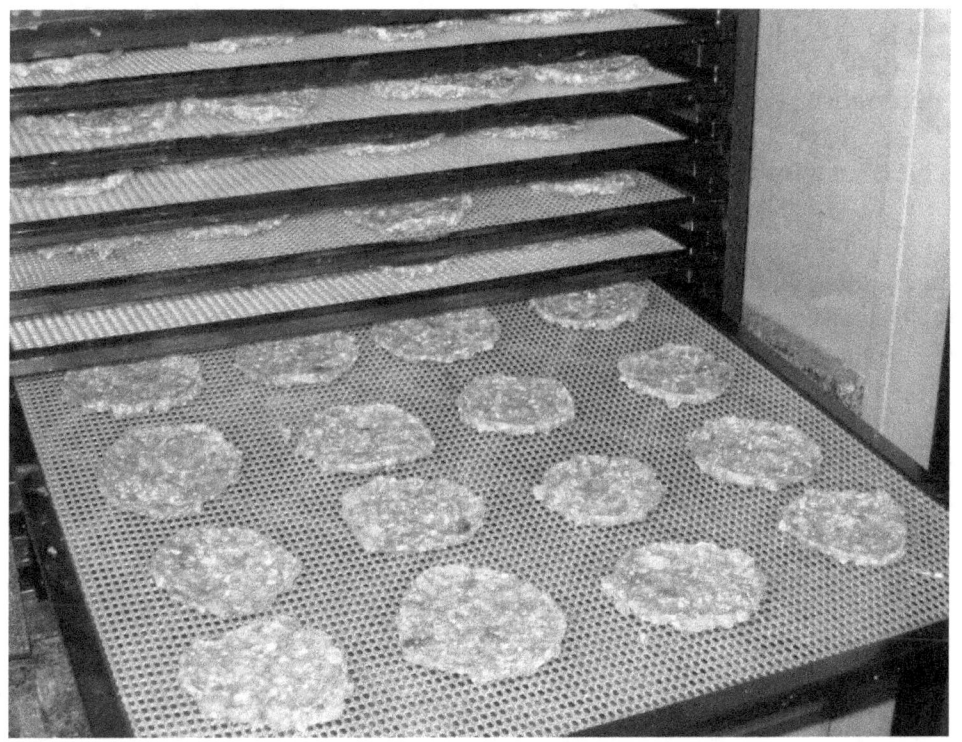

Ingredients:
3 cups fresh raw corn kernels (cut 'em off the cob, of course!) (no canned corn please!)
1 1/2 cups yellow pepper
3/4 cup flax seed (finely ground, so use ground flax seed or grind some whole flax seeds yourself in a coffee grinder)
1 tablespoon lime juice (fresh) (you could probably use lemon if you have to)
1 tablespoon chili powder
1 teaspoon sea salt

Preparation Time 10 min
Wait Time 10 hours

Total Time 10 hours 10 min
Serving Size Varies
Shelf Life Eat immediately
Equipment Food Processor   Dehydrator

Directions:
1. Throw the corn and yellow pepper in the food processor. Process until almost smooth.

2. Add the remaining ingredients and process in your food processor until nicely blended for cracker/chip type texture. Don't over-process. Note: Flax seeds act as the binding agent (keeps this recipe stuck together) so don't omit the ground flax for God's sake! This raw corn chip recipe needs flax!

3. Throw the mixture in your dehydrator. As per the above photo, circles are the easiest to lay out in your dehydrator. But you can also do a whole sheet and then cut or snap them when they're partially dehydrated.

4. I usually dehydrate at 115 degrees for the first hour and then lower to 105 for the remaining time frame. Check them after four hours. If possible, flip them over and dehydrate for another four hours or so.

Remember, dehydrating is an art and depends on lots of variables. So just check on 'em every once in a while.

3.6 Salads

Chopped Salad

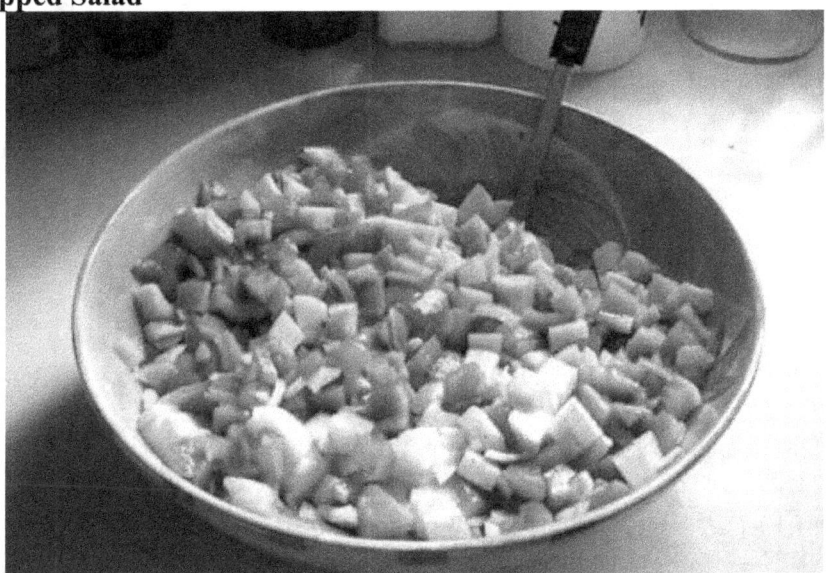

Preparation Time: 15 minutes
Servings: 6-8

Ingredients:
2 medium cucumbers
2 large red tomatoes
1 large red onion
2 medium green peppers
5 tablespoons lemon juice
1/2 cup oil Salt and pepper, to taste

Directions:
1) Wash and then chop vegetables into tiny little cubes. Add to a large bowl and stir in oil and lemon juice. Season to taste. Chill for about 2 hours before serving and enjoy.

Tomato & Olive Salad

Serves 4

Ingredients:
4 parts cherry tomatoes
1 part olives
Raw extra virgin olive oil
2 tablespoons lemon juice
Pepper
Basil to taste
Rugola lettuce or other greens (optional)

Directions:

Break the tomatoes so that the juice comes out (best in a cup so juice won't spill) Combine the tomatoes and olives in a bowl. Add the olive oil, lemon juice and pepper. Toss. Just before dinner, add the basil and Rugola. Most olives are salty so that you don't need extra salt. In case you find raw olive that don't have salt on them yet, then you might like to add some Himalayan sea salt.

RAW TACO SALAD

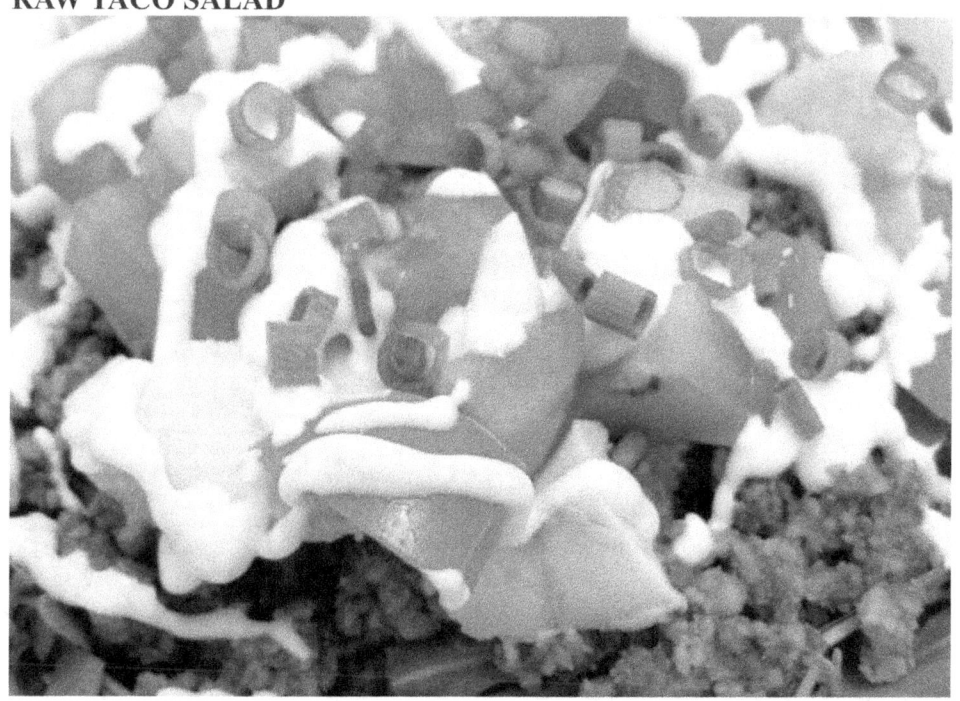

Ingredients:
Walnut Taco Meat (4 serves)

1 cup (150g) walnuts
½ packed cup (50g) sun-dried tomatoes, soaked 2-8h and drained
½ tsp cumin
¼ tsp garlic powder
⅛-1/4 tsp salt (adjust to taste)
pinch chili (or more if you like it hot)
pinch cayenne pepper

Cashew Sour Cream (12 serves)

1 cup (140g) cashews, soaked 1-2h (soaking optional)

scant ¼ cup (55g) lemon juice
¼ tsp salt
⅓ cup (85g) water
⅔ cup (95g) ice

Salad (1 serve)

2 cups rocket (arugula)
¼ cup Walnut Taco Meat (see above)
½ avocado
1 med tomato
1 tsbp Cashew Sour Cream (see above)
1 tbsp spring onion, sliced

Instructions:
1) Cover the sun-dried tomatoes in water and leave to soak for 2 to 8 hours. Drain.

2) Process all of the walnut taco meat ingredients in a food processor until well combined, but still chunky.

3) Blend all of the cashew sour cream ingredients in a blender until smooth and creamy.

4) Assemble salad ingredients in a large bowl (one per person),

5) serve and eat.

Avocado Nectarine Salad

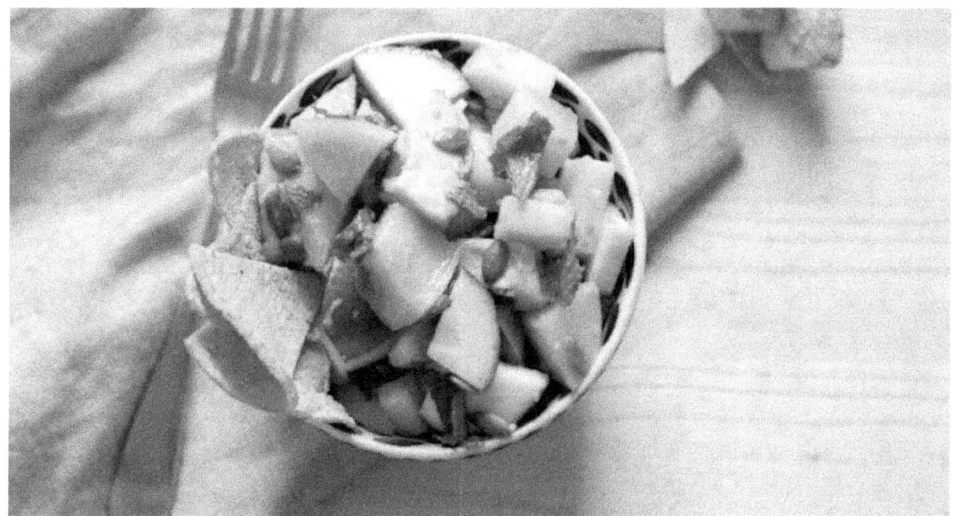

Ingredients:

- 1 nectarine
- 1 avocado
- 1/3 medium zucchini
- 1/3 medium cucumber, peeled
- 2 Tbsp. pumpkin seeds
- 10 mint leaves, torn into little pieces
- Juice from half a lime
- Dash of salt

Instructions:

1. Chop the nectarine, avocado, zucchini, and cucumber into small cubes and place in a bowl.

2. Add the pumpkin seeds, mint leaves, lime juice, and dash of salt.

3. Mix everything together and enjoy!

Blueberry Mango Salad with Ginger Tahini Dressing

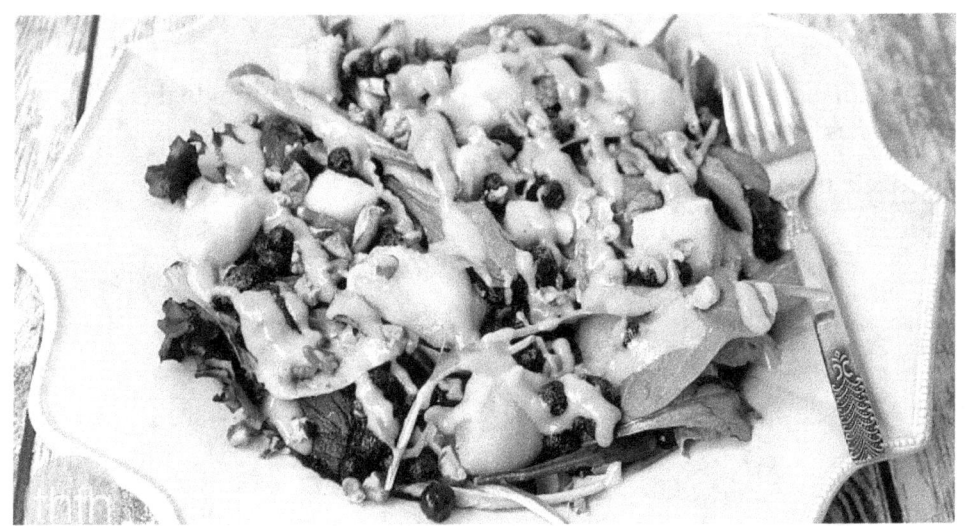

Ingredients:

- 2 handfuls organic spring salad mix
- 1/2 cup organic blueberries
- 1/2 cup organic mango (cubed)
- 1/4 cup organic pecans

Ingredients:

- 2 tablespoons organic raw tahini
- 1/2 - 1 tablespoon organic agave
- 1/8 teaspoon organic ground ginger
- 2 tablespoons purified/filtered water

Instructions:

1. Add all ingredients to a small bowl and stir until well combined.

2. Adjust sweetener to your preference and water if you prefer a thinner consistency.

Instructions:

1. Add 2 handfuls of spring salad mix to your plate and sprinkle the blueberries, diced mango and pecans over the top.

2. Drizzle the Tahini Ginger Dressing over the top. Enjoy!

Citrus Fruit Winter Salad

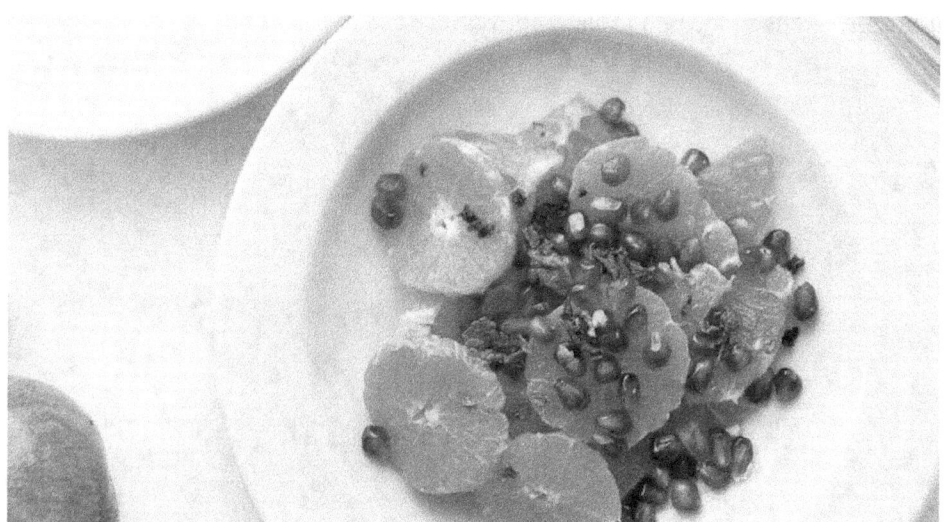

Ingredients:

- 1 pink grapefruit

- 2-3 clementines

- 1/2 pomegranate, deseeded

- a few leaves of fresh mint

Instructions:

1. Wash and peel off the skins of the fruit. Cut the grapefruit into chunks and slice the clementines into slices so it looks pretty in a wide bowl.

2. To deseed the pomegranate, submerge into a bowl of cool water and cut and pull apart the pieces while the fruit is submerged in the water. Then, drain the seeds in a calendar and enjoy!

Dilly Curry-Tahini Salad

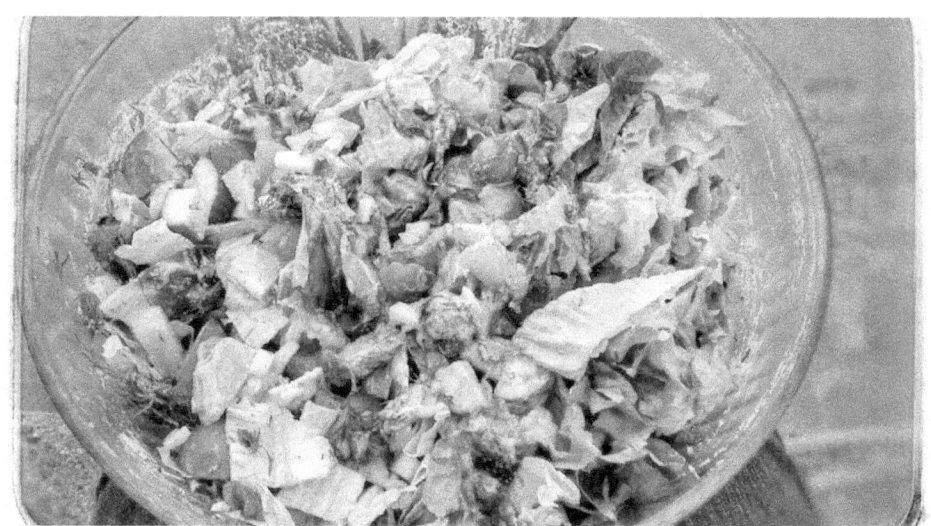

Ingredients:

- 1 head of lettuce, chopped
- 2 cups cherry tomatoes, chopped
- 1/4 sweet white onion, diced
- 2 spring onions, chopped
- 1/2 bell pepper, chopped
- 2 Persian cucumbers, chopped

Dressing:

- 2 tbsp organic tahini
- 1 tbsp chia seeds
- 1/2 medium zucchini

- 1 tbsp curry powder
- 1 tbsp onion powder
- 1/4 teaspoon Himalayan salt
- juice of 1/2 lemon
- a splash of water
- 2-3 tablespoons chopped fresh dill, or to taste

Instructions

Salad:

1. Chop all of the vegetables and place them in a bowl.

Dressing:

1. Combine all ingredients besides dill in a blender with just enough water to blend.

2. Blend until completely smooth. If you are not using a high speed blender, mill your chia seeds in a coffee grinder first so that they are broken down.

Place in a bowl and mix with the fresh chopped dill. Mix with the salad and enjoy.

Late Summer Garden Salad

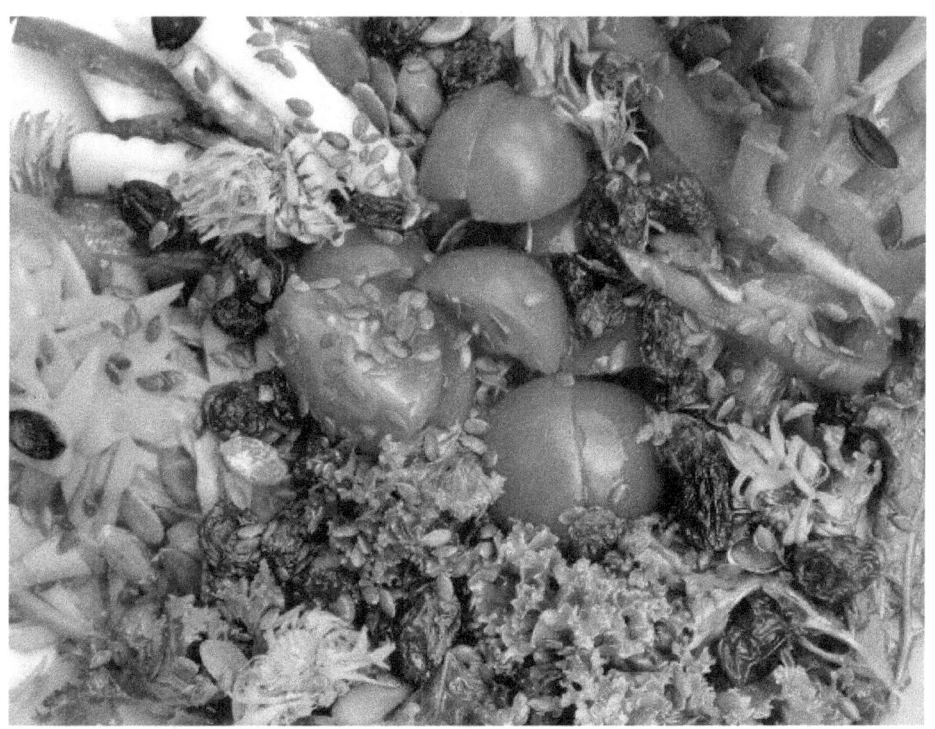

Ingredients:

a few handfuls of washed and chopped kale

half a red bell pepper

one carrot

half a cucumber

a few cherry tomatoes

2 tbsp raisins

1 tbsp pumpkin seeds

1 tsp flax seeds

1 tbsp flax seed oil (cold-pressed)

a few edible flowers

himalayan sea salt

Instructions:

1) Add the chopped kale to a bowl.

2) Slice the other vegetables and add to the salad.

3) Drizzle over raisins, pumpkin- and flaxseeds, flaxseed oil, the edible flowers and some himalayan sea salt.

Mango Salad with Agave-Lime Dressing

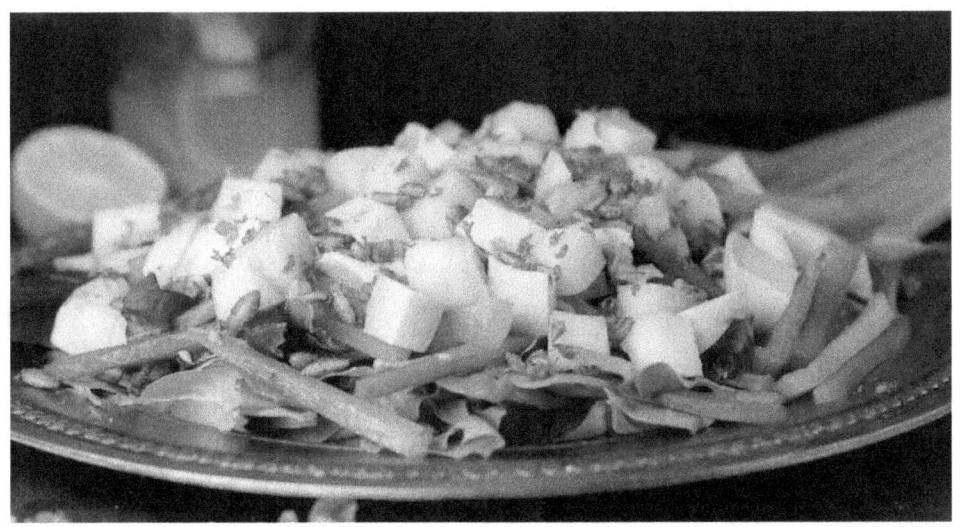

Ingredients:

"Honey"-Lime Dressing:
- 3/4 cup olive oil
- 4 1/2 tablespoons fresh lime juice
- 1 1/2 tablespoons agave
- 1 teaspoon mustard flakes
- 1/2 teaspoon crushed red pepper flakes (more if you want!)
- 1 large clove garlic, minced
- sea salt and pepper, to taste

Salad:
- 11oz mixed greens
- 1 mango, diced
- 1 avocado, peeled and diced

- 1 red bell pepper, sliced
- 1 orange bell pepper, sliced
- 1/4 cup minced fresh parsley
- 1/3 cup raw or sprouted pepitas
- Agave-lime dressing, to taste

Instructions:

1. In a large bowl, toss all salad ingredients together dressing is evenly distributed. Enjoy!

Rainbow Noodle Salad with Pesto

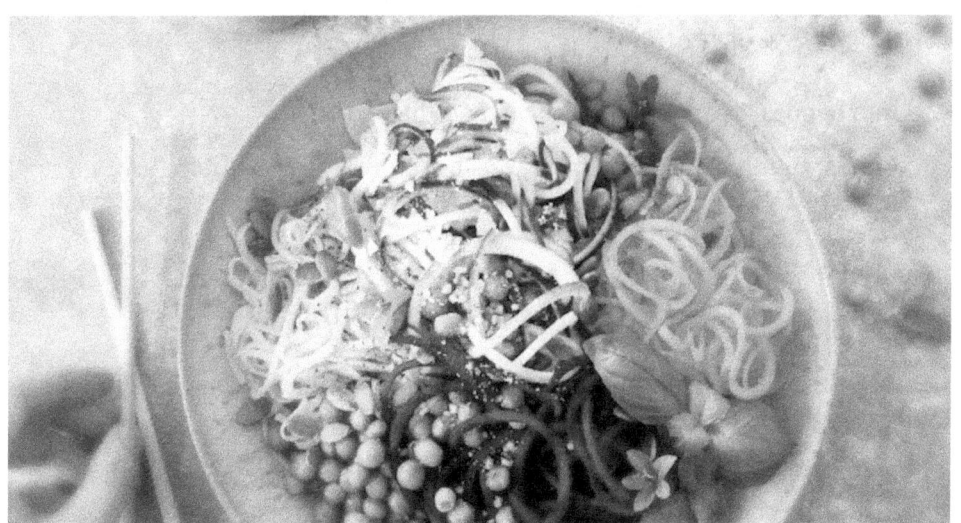

Ingredients:

Pea Pumpkin Seed Pesto:

- 1 cup peas, fresh or frozen and thawed
- 2 large handfuls fresh herbs (I used basil + oregano)
- 4 tablespoons pumpkin seeds
- 2 tablespoons extra virgin olive oil
- 1 tablespoon lime (or lemon) juice
- 1 tablespoon Shiro miso & nutritional yeast each (optional, for a salty 'cheesy' flavor)
- ½ teaspoon Himalayan crystal salt or sea salt
- Black pepper & turmeric, to taste (optional)

Rainbow Noodle Salad:

- 1 ½ Cups of spiralized vegetables (zucchinni)
- 2 large carrots
- 1 large beetroot
- 1 large handful peas, fresh or frozen and thawed
- Toppings: pumpkin seeds, almond, cashew, fresh herbs, edible flowers

Instructions:

Pea Pumpkin Seed Pesto:

1. Add your peas, herbs, pumpkin seeds, olive oil, lime juice and salt to a food processor fitted with an S-blade. Process until creamy.

2. I also like to add black pepper and turmeric because they have really strong anti-inflammatory properties + miso and nutritional yeast for a salty 'cheesy' flavor.

Rainbow Noodle Salad:

1. Use a spiralizer to turn your zucchini, carrots and beetroot into noodles. If you're using organic veggies, you can leave the skin on for extra minerals - just make sure to rinse them well. If not, it's best to peel the vegetables.

2. Combine the vegetables noodles in a bowl. I like to serve the pesto on the side so you can add as much or as little as you want.

3. For garnish, I used pumpkin seeds, almond, cashew, basil and oregano (the same herbs I used for the pesto) and a few edible flowers.

Notes • This pesto will stay fresh for at least 3 days in an airtight container in the fridge.

SPICY ZOODLE BOWL

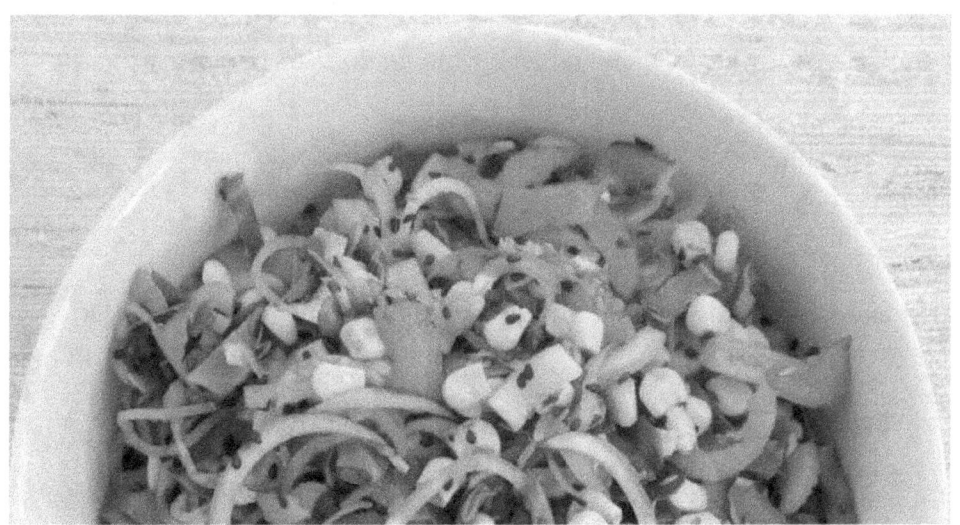

Ingredients:

Main Ingredients:

- 1 large zucchini, spiralized or peeled
- 2 large carrots, spiralized or peeled
- 1 red bell pepper, sliced thin (any color is good)
- 1 cup purple cabbage, chopped into small strips
- 1 cup fresh corn (optional)
- 1/2 cup celery, chopped small
- 1/4 cup fresh cilantro, chopped
- 2-3 tablespoons sesame seeds

Spicy Dressing:

1-inch piece of fresh ginger, peel removed

1/4- 1/2 inch chunk of jalapeno, depending on your spiciness liking)

1/2 of an avocado,

fresh juice from 1 lime

1/4 - 1/3 cup of water, depending on how thick/thin you prefer your dressing)

2 teaspoons agave

1/2 tablespoon raw, unrefined, organic coconut oil

1/4 teaspoon fine-grain sea salt, pepper, to taste

Optional add-ins: cashews, peanuts, edamame, green onions, hemp hearts

Instructions:

1. Spiralize or peel zucchini and carrots.

2. Add to a large bowl along with the red pepper, purple cabbage, corn, celery, cilantro and sesame seeds. Mix well.

FOR THE DRESSING:

1. In a blender, combine all of the dressing ingredients and blend until smooth. Pour dressing over salad, mix well and serve!

Summer Cabbage Corn Slaw

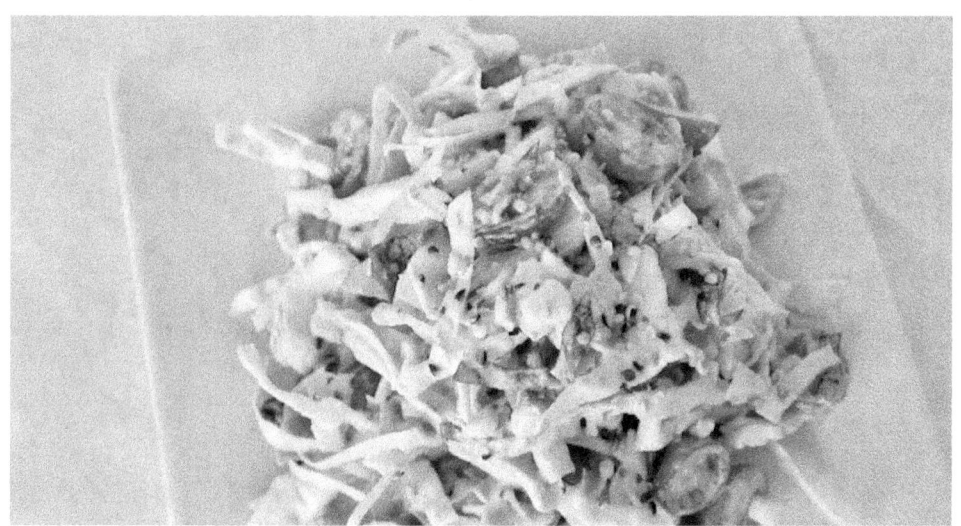

Ingredients:

- 1 small head cabbage, shredded
- 1 cup fresh sweet corn
- 3 scallions, sliced
- 1 cup cherry tomatoes, halved
- 1/4 cup fresh basil, chopped
- 3 Tbs raw shelled hemp seeds

Dressing:

- 1/2 cup sweet corn
- 3 Tbsp raw walnut butter
- 1/4 cup filtered water
- 1/4 cup apple cider vinegar
- 1 medjool date, pitted

- 2 Tbsp nutritional yeast (optional)
- 1 clove garlic
- 1 tsp turmeric
- sea salt to taste

Instructions:

1. In a large bowl, combine all of the veggies and basil.

2. In a high speed blender, combine all of the dressing ingredients and blend until smooth and well combined.

3. Toss with the salad, and the hemp seeds. Serve!

Zesty Kale Cucumber Caesar Salad

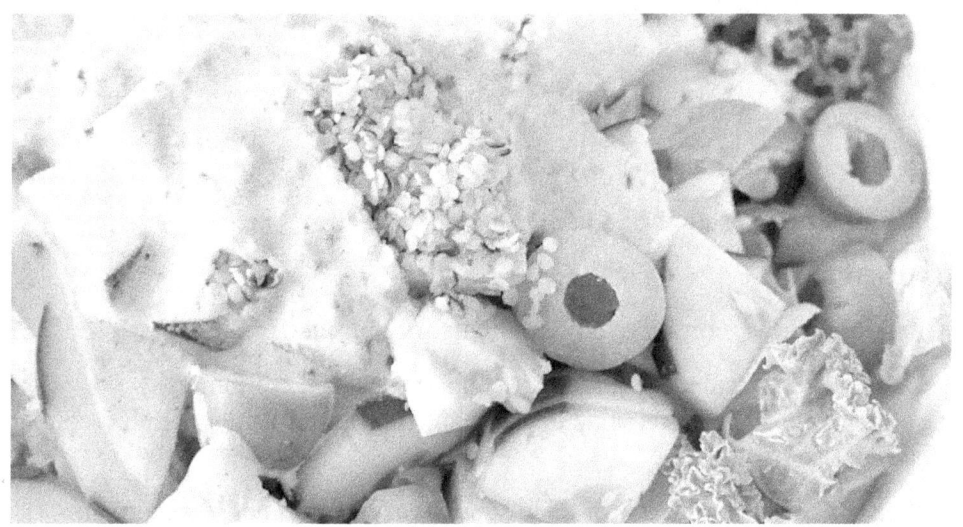

Ingredients:

Salad:

- 3-4 curly kale leaves, torn into pieces
- 1 bunch of romaine hearts, chopped
- 2/3 cucumber, quartered
- 1/4 cup green olives, sliced
- 1/4 cup hemp seeds
- optional add-ins: capers(Capers are the pickled flower buds of a shrub that grows all over the Mediterranean), pine nuts.

Vegan Caesar Dressing:

- 1/3 cup hemp seeds
- 1/3 cup water
- 1 tablespoon mustard flakes

- 1/2 tablespoon raw apple cider vinegar
- 1/2 teaspoon minced garlic
- 1/2 teaspoon agave nectar
- 1/4 teaspoon sea salt
- 1/4 teaspoon black pepper
- 2 tablespoons fresh lemon juice

Instructions:

1. In a large bowl, combine all ingredients for the salad and mix.

2. Using a hand immersion blender or food processor, combine all ingredients for the Caesar salad dressing and blend until smooth and creamy. Makes 1 cup worth.

3. Pour dressing over salad (or keep separate if you planned for leftovers). Enjoy!

3.7 Smoothies and juices

Vegetable Juice Recipe #1
Carrot Juice

Here's my favorite carrot juice recipe. I make this juice almost every morning. Very quick and easy:

Ingredients:

1 lbs large carrots (washed and peeled)
1/2 lemon (peeled)
few green leafs such as red lettuce or carrot greens
1 apple

Directions:

Put all ingredients in your juicer. (A centrifuge juicer is easiest for carrots.) Mix. Drink immediately.

I peel the carrot for taste (otherwise it tastes too earthy). I find this recipe sweet enough, but if you're a beginner juicer or have a sweet tooth, add an apple for extra sweetness.

The health benefits of carrot juice? It provides Vitamin A, B Vitamins, Vitamin E and many minerals (including calcium). Great for pregnant and nursing mothers, eyesight, bones and teeth, liver and nails, skin and hair as well as helping in breast and skin cancer prevention.

Vegetable Juice Recipe #2
Tomato Juice

Are you looking for the best of all tomato juice recipes! This one is! You can juice the tomatoes in a juicer but if you have a high speed blender - such as a Vitamix or Blendec Blender - and you like more "body" to your juice, you might like to use the blender in stead.

Here's the recipe for your own V8 juice: quick, easy and yummy!

Ingredients:

3 cups chopped tomatoes
1 stalk celery
1 cucumber
3 drops stevia (optional)
1/2 teaspoon himalaya sea salt
pepper
cayenne pepper

Directions:

Juice the tomatoes, celery, cucumber in your juicer.
Add drops stevia if you like a sweeter taste, salt, pepper and cayenne pepper to taste.

If you like you can also add a 1/4 onion, fresh oregano and basil and red bell pepper.

Mmmmm so good!

Vegetable Juice Recipe #3
Spinach Juice

This juice recipe is perfect for starters of veggie juicing. It's soft and sweet. Very tasty. Not bitter or strong at all.

Ingredients:
1 bunch spinach
2 apples
1/2 lemon, peeled (optional)

Directions:
Put all ingredients in your juicer. A twin gear juicer such as the Green Star Juicer is best for extracting greens.
Mix well and enjoy.
You don't have to add the lemon, it's good enough without it. But I just love lemon, so I always add a little.

Vegetable Juice Recipe #4
Cabbage Juice

Cabbage juice is known for its ability to heal peptic ulcers. It's is full of vitamin K, C, fiber, manganese, B6, Folic Acid, Omega 3 fatty acids, calcium, phytonutrients and anti-oxidants. And very low in calories.

Cabbage is so good for you. Recent studies show that people who eat most cabbage have a significantly lower risk of colon, lung, breast and prostate cancer. Even compared to other people that eat lots of veggies.

Red cabbage has even more nutrients and protects against Alzheimer's disease (Food Science and Technology).

Juicing cabbage is a superb way to get the best out of your cabbage. Cabbage provides anti-carcinogenic glucosinolates (anti cancer fighters). When you cook cabbage, you kill the special myrosinase enzyme that makes the cabbage so healing, thus making cabbage less effective as anti cancer food.

Drinking it straight might be a little too much in the beginning. Then, simply mix it with carrot juice. Start with juicing carrots. Every day add some cabbage leafs until you're used to the taste. (The taste isn't that strong.) You may also try other cruciferous family members of cabbage such as kale, broccoli, and collard greens.

Jamba Juice Recipe
Wheat Grass Juice w Orange

Jamba Juice has a great wheat grass juice recipe: They serve their wheat grass with a slice of orange. I really like that idea. It makes the wheat grass a little fancier. And in case you don't like the taste of wheat grass - after finishing your juice, you can take a bite of the orange!

Wheat grass is so good for you! It has most of the vitamins and minerals needed for human health. It is a complete protein with about 30 enzymes. It has up to 70% chlorophyll (which builds the blood). It's an excellent source of calcium, iron, magnesium, phosphorus, potassium, and zinc. And it's one of the best alkaline foods.

Raw Vegan Smoothie Recipe

Ingredients:
1 Whole Coconut
2 Tbl Cacao Nibs
2 Tbl Maca
1 Tbl Lucuma
1 Tbl Mesquite
Favorite Fruit
Agave
Sea Salt

How to Prepare:
1. Place coconut meat and coconut water in your high speed blender.
2. Add the rest of the ingredients.
3. Blend until smooth.

Chocolate Smoothie Recipe

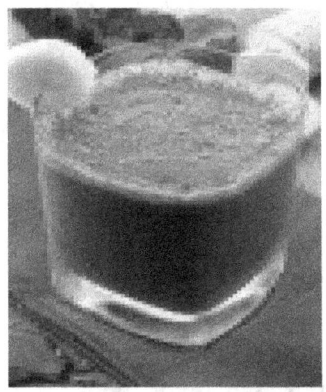

Do you feel the august heat? Treat yourself to a delicious chocolate smoothie recipe. A fabulous and healthy summer drink. (Vegan and raw.)
I just love chocolate. And knowing that you can make a scrumptious vegan raw food smoothie that is actually good for you, just makes me so happy. Life is good!

Ingredients:
Serves 2

2 bananas
1 tablespoon hemp seed
1 bag of frozen blueberries (about 250 gram or 1 cup)
1/2 teaspoon of liquid stevia
Pure water
2 teaspoons of raw chocolate (powder or nibs)
1 teaspoon raw carob powder (optional)
1/2 teaspoon of green powder (optional)
1/2 teaspoon of mesquite (optional)
1 teaspoon of lucuma (optional)
1/2 teaspoon of cinnamon powder
pinch of cayenne pepper

Directions:

Put all ingredients in a high speed blender. Add enough pure water so that all ingredients are covered. Blend well.

You may want to add a little more water if the smoothie gets too thick. You may blend longer if you find the smoothie too cold.

Tips

Instead of hemp seeds you can also use cashew nuts or coconut meat.
You don't have to use blueberries, but I really like the taste of them in combination with the chocolate.
I always add a bunch of or super foods to this smoothie for mineralization and extra nutrition. Don't be scared by the number. I just use whatever super foods I have available at home. Sometimes all of them, sometimes none. The ones listed above just go really well with the chocolate.

If you'd like a stronger chocolate taste, you can add some more chocolate powder of course. I then recommend to add a little agave for taste to this chocolate smoothie recipe. (Together with the stevia which you use to sweeten it).

CHAPTER 4

MENU PLANS

4.1 Simple, no equipment needed menus

In the following pages you will find several examples of meal plans. These are meant as samples and can be mixed and matched as much as you would like to do. At the end of this book I mentioned several other books from other authors with excellent meal plans as well.

SAMPLE MENU PLAN #1

RAW DIET BREAKFAST MEALS:

Oatmeal: Soak whole oats overnight, warm, add pinch of salt and Sucanat to taste. Fruit salad: Many recipes into one with endless combinations. Chop your choice of fruit, add vanilla raw yogurt (recipe included in next chapter), or scoop of frozen pineapple juice concentrate, or coconut milk. You can also add shredded dried or fresh coconut. Sprout bread: Found in health stores. Baked on very low heat, sweet with cake-like texture. My favorite is Manna Raisin Carrot. Warning: very high in calories, easy to overeat. Great raw food if anticipating high energy output. Raw power protein cereal: Blend the following in a coffee grinder until powdered: 1 tbsp. flax seeds, 2 tbsp. sesame seeds, 2 tbsp. sunflower seeds and 5 almonds. (of course all raw) Add raw agave and small amounts of hot water (not boiling). Mix until desired consistency. Slice banana on top with a sprinkle of Sucanat or raw agave. Can also add raw pumpkin seeds or replace bananas with raisins. Mix and match to make your own blend. A highly concentrated, filling food. Eat slowly, chew well. Homemade raw trail mix: Two or three handfuls of this concentrated food with fruit provide a great start for the day. Here are some suggested raw ingredients: chopped dates, raisins, dried apricots, cashews, sesame seeds, filberts, pumpkin seeds, walnuts, shredded coconut, chopped figs, dried currants, dried banana chips, almonds, sunflower seeds, brazil nuts, whole oats, dried apple. Makes a convenient fast food.

RAW DIET LUNCH MEALS:

Avocado dressing for cut veggies. Here is my favorite recipe: 1 ripe avocado 1 tbsp. agave ½ tbsp. lemon juice 1 tsp. garlic powder ½ tsp. onion power sea salt to taste.

Blender smoothies: Many recipes blended into one. Suggestions are your choice of any fruit. Try flavoring with cinnamon, raw soy yogurt, coconut milk, or almond butter. For extra caloric punch add avocado, figs, dates and raisins. A handful of ice cubes will thicken into a refreshing drink on hot days. Banana almond butter dip: Easy and fast. Stand at counter, add small dab of almond butter after each banana bite. Cleanup is a peel and knife. Done like dinner!

Raw corn: Barefoot in kitchen, husk a cob of corn and eat. You have got to try this, it tastes great. No salt, butter, muss or fuss.

Romaine and nori roll-ups: Diced avocado, alfalfa sprouts, a nori (edible seaweed) sheet, chopped green onion, shredded carrot, romaine, diced tomato. Mix together all but nori and lettuce. Place a nori sheet on a romaine lettuce leaf and top with a scoop of the vegetable mixture. Roll up and secure the bundle together with toothpick.

Nut milk shake:
Add a half-cup of water to raw cashews and blend until smooth.
Add 2 more cups water
2 tbsp. Agave
½ tsp. vanilla extract
5 ice cubes and continue blending. Very filling.

RAW DIET SUPPER MEALS:

Fruit and nut salad: Mix diced apples, diced celery, grapes and chopped walnuts. Puree bananas and pour over, stir, and enjoy. Sprinkle Sucanat on top. Versatile veggie salad combos: There is a wealth of raw materials you can combine to produce a filling, delicious salad. All manner of greens and sprouts, topped with raw nuts and salad dressings homemade from cold-pressed oil. While eating, just think of the cleansing, healing nutrients you are feeding every cell. Carrot-raisin salad:3 lb. Carrots, 1 cup of raisins, ½ can frozen pineapple concentrate. Finely grate carrots, add pineapple concentrate and raisins. Allow to stand in refrigerator overnight.

Raw tomato soup:

Blend roma tomatoes with your favorite spices. Warm and eat or add favorite vegetables. Suggested additions: garlic cloves, basil, onion, sea salt, flaked yeast, simulated chicken base Fresh veggie juice: For a challenge, try just having a few glasses of veggie juice as a supper meal. A great way to encourage detoxification during a good night's sleep.

RAW DIET SNACKS:

Fruit, nuts, dried fruit: A bag of pre-washed, peeled fruit, raw nuts or dried fruit in the passenger seat is a great drive-through deterrent.

Sweet potato pudding: Blend ½ cantaloupe, ½ sweet potato, 3 tbsp. sucanat, 5 ice cubes and pinch of cinnamon. The flavor is somewhere between pumpkin pie and chocolate pudding. Great treat.

SAMPLE MENU PLAN #2:

Raw Food Breakfast:
Personal Development guru Steven Pavlina began his documented raw foods diet with this enormous breakfast of fruits and greens:
1 Green Smoothie:
2 Bananas
2 cups of mixed greens
1 cup of water
8 Clementines
Fruit Plate: of grapes, 2 celery stalks and a sliced mango
Fruit Salad: 2 bananas, strawberries, blackberries and blueberries

At over 1000 calories, this is a very large breakfast, and many raw fooders would prefer to cut it by about half. Many people simply snack all morning. Raw Foods Lunch Pavlina began incorporating more greens into his diet that was so high in fruits. An example of one of his Raw foods lunches starts with a larger salad: 96g of mixed greens 72g Avocado 8g Lime juice 2 carrots 2 celery sticks Other lunch examples are as simple as a large salad with several pieces of fruit, fresh or dried, complemented with nuts and juices. Smoothies are also a popular meal of choice. Raw Foods Dinner

According to Vegetarian.com, people that adhere to this diet claim to feel improved overall health and more energy and well being. They promote combining foods to get a well-rounded balance of nutrients. A healthy dinner could be the following: Large spinach salad mixed with romaine lettuce 1 cucumber 1 tomato 1 green onion 1 orange water or fruit juice Many people tend to find combinations of foods that go well together and stimulate their taste buds.

More often than not, experimenting is half the fun. Don't be afraid of fresh vegetables and nontraditional nuts and seeds. Snack Attack Raw foods snacking is encouraged. "Grazing" or eating small amounts of foods like various seeds, nuts, fruits and veggies keeps you full in between meals.

SAMPLE MENU PLAN #3:

Sample Menus for averaging a 2,000 calorie diet.

Menu 1:
Breakfast: Smoothie with 5 bananas and 2 mangoes.
Lunch: 5 oranges and 3 grapefruit.
Snack: 1/4 watermelon.
Dinner: Salad with 1 head romaine, 1 cup spinach, 1 red pepper, 1/2 avocado, 2 roma tomatoes, 1 cucumber, 1/2 cup corn.

Menu 2:
Breakfast: 1/4 watermelon.
Snack: Fruit salad with 3 oranges, 3 tangerines, 1 grapefruit.
Lunch: Salad with 1 head romaine, 1/2 avocado, 1 tomato, 5 unsalted olives
Snack: Smoothie with 5 bananas, 2 cups strawberries.

Dinner: Salad with 6 cups spinach, 1 red pepper, 1 ounce almonds, 1 cucumber.

Menu 3:
Breakfast: 1 honeydew melon.
Lunch: 10 oranges/
Dinner: 10 oz baby greens, 2 stalks celery, 2 cups grape tomatoes, 1 ounce cashews, 1 cup carrots.
Snack: Smoothie with 3 bananas, 2 cups pineapple.

Menu 4:
Breakfast: 3 apples, 3 pears.
Lunch: 6 mangoes.
Snack: Baby carrots and guacamole made with 1 avocado, diced tomatoes and red pepper, cilantro, and lime.
Dinner: Salad with 10 oz iceberg, 2 tomatoes, 1/2 cup corn, 1 cup strawberries, 4 dates.

Menu 5:
Breakfast: Fruit salad with 2 cups red grapes, 2 bananas, 1 orange, 1 grapefruit, 1 apple.
Lunch: lettuce wraps
Snack: 8 bananas
Dinner: Zucchini pasta with raw marinara

CHAPTER 5

ACTUAL CASE HISTORIES OF HEALING THROUGH A RAW, VEGAN DIET

Below are a couple of case histories from my patients who utilized a raw, vegan diet as a part of their healing protocol. One deals with long term heavy metal poisoning as a sculptor and a welder. The other patient presented with stage 4 cancer and was told she only had about six months to live without chemotherapy.

5.1 Case History #1 – Betsy – Heavy Metal Toxicity

I know from experience that this is not most patient's favorite subject, one of diet. As Doctor Christopher once stated, **"Talk to a friend about their diet and you will lose a friend"**. Sadly, I have seen this so many times. But it is a simple fact that you are what you eat and if you eat dead food it will not produce life within your body.

One of the most prevalent conditions in America today as well as in other industrialized nations is heavy metal toxicity. It is found in the food, the air, the soil, cigarette smoking and in the cloths we wear. Pharmaceuticals are filled with them such as mercury, aluminum, cadmium, lead and arsenic.

Some time back a 47 year old female patient came into our clinic complaining of a number of autoimmune type reactions as well as a serious candida and mold infection. During her intake we found that she was a potter and sculptor who made extensive use of glazing.

Heavy metals can be found in the clay itself as well as the chemicals used for glazing. Her home also had a very serious mold problem. Her blood work showed infections and a hair analysis showed extensive heavy metals as can be seen by the following lab result:

		TOXIC METALS		PERCENTILE
		RESULT mg/g	REFERENCE INTERVAL	68th 95th
Aluminum	(Al)	8.1	< 7.0	
Antimony	(Sb)	0.12	< 0.050	
Arsenic	(As)	0.048	< 0.060	
Barium	(Ba)	4.0	< 2.0	
Beryllium	(Be)	< 0.01	< 0.020	
Bismuth	(Bi)	0.096	< 2.0	
Cadmium	(Cd)	0.12	< 0.050	
Lead	(Pb)	5.6	< 0.60	
Mercury	(Hg)	0.15	< 0.80	
Platinum	(Pt)	< 0.003	< 0.005	
Thallium	(Tl)	< 0.001	< 0.002	
Thorium	(Th)	0.002	< 0.002	
Uranium	(U)	0.014	< 0.060	
Nickel	(Ni)	0.29	< 0.30	
Silver	(Ag)	5.5	< 0.15	
Tin	(Sn)	1.1	< 0.30	
Titanium	(Ti)	0.57	< 0.70	
Total Toxic Representation				

She was very high in Antimony, Barium, Lead, Nickel and Silver. These metals are notorious for wiping out the intestinal flora and bringing bout a severe candida overgrowth, thereby compromising the immune system. This left her open to so many other co-infections such as mold and other bacterial types. Her original presenting complaints included candida and hormonal imbalances.

We stated her off with our standard candida cleanse, mentioned earlier in this document. This utilized a vegan diet due to it's low inflammatory nature and one low in natural sugar. She had to avoid all sugars and alcohol, even fruits for at least 18 days as well as use holistic medications for killing the candida, such as Black walnut and Pau'd Arco. We keep the bowels moving to help eliminate the dead yeast.

By the end of the 18 days she noticed a marked improvement in her thinking and level of energy. She proceeded to have the home cleaned out from the mold while we treated her for the mold in lungs, again, using the above mold and yeast formulas, but at a much lower dosage and for several months. She remained on the vegan diet as it is well established that the fiber and anti-oxidants and other chemicals in the plants help chelate the heavy metals from her body.

At this time we also prescribed a natural heavy metal formula called Dr. Christopher's Bugle Heavy Metal Formula. It utilizes Bugleweed, a known herb with a very strong history of success for removing heavy metals from the body. She remained on this program for at least six months. As each month passed on the program she felt her health improving which we conformed with blood work demonstrating the infections were disappearing. We finally ran another heavy metal hair test six months later. The surprising results are shown below:

TOXIC METALS		RESULT mg/g	REFERENCE INTERVAL	PERCENTILE 68th 95th
Aluminum	(Al)	3.6	< 7.0	
Antimony	(Sb)	0.035	< 0.050	
Arsenic	(As)	0.048	< 0.060	
Barium	(Ba)	1.5	< 2.0	
Beryllium	(Be)	< 0.01	< 0.020	
Bismuth	(Bi)	0.013	< 2.0	
Cadmium	(Cd)	0.046	< 0.050	
Lead	(Pb)	1.2	< 0.60	
Mercury	(Hg)	0.08	< 0.80	
Platinum	(Pt)	< 0.003	< 0.005	
Thallium	(Tl)	< 0.001	< 0.002	
Thorium	(Th)	0.001	< 0.002	
Uranium	(U)	0.020	< 0.060	
Nickel	(Ni)	0.12	< 0.30	
Silver	(Ag)	1.4	< 0.15	
Tin	(Sn)	0.14	< 0.30	
Titanium	(Ti)	0.34	< 0.70	
Total Toxic Representation				

As you can see from the above lab, the heavy metals showed a marked improvement which was mirrored in her improved energy levels, thinking and memory abilities and a total lack of bronchial and sinus issues.

She remains vegan, high raw, to this day and is a shining example of a healthy and happy individual. We are all very proud of her.

5.2 Case History #2 - Kim – Inoperable colon/appendix cancer

The cancer rate statistics in the year 1900 was 1 out 50 would have this disease sometime in their lifetime. By the 1970's, the start of the "war on Cancer", the rate was up to 1 out of 10. Today it has grown to 1 out 2 people in the United States will experience cancer sometime in their lifetime. Needless to say, the war on cancer is not being won.

At our clinic we have seen many. Many cases of cancer and the number of patients presenting this illness is on the rise within our practice. One particular case stands out as one of my patients to have had the joy and privilege to know.

She was a 59 year old woman who originally came to the clinic to be treated for psoriasis. During her initial appointment she asked if I would check on lump on her lower right abdomen. I told her I would be happy to check. She stated her other doctor had checked and dismissed it as a simply fatty deposit but her heart told her different. When we were going over her treatment plan for the psoriasis I lead her and her husband into the exam room.

I have been around quite a bit of cancer in my 20+ years of practice and as soon as I palpated the area I knew what it was. But, I kept the traditional poker face and suggested we check with ultrasound. We have ultrasound at the clinic so it was a simple matter of setting the machine up and within five minutes we were scanning the site. Her entire abdominal cavity was full of what appeared to be tumors and acites (fluid filled pockets often caused by cancer in the bowels and appendix).

The poker face was gone and she could see there was some concern. I requested we get some blood work done to get a better idea. She agreed and when the lab results came in it confirmed a 95% likelihood of cancer. She became very upset with her doctor dismissing her since at this point she had lost two months of possible treatment time. She returned to them and showed them our results. At this point the other doctor panicked and reran all of my tests and found the same results. The final diagnosis was colon and appendix cancer with Pseudomyxoma peritonei (PMP) She was staged at stage four.

Or course, the recommended treatment plan from them was to surgically bulk the cancer and to run a very risky chemo therapy treatment that requires extensive blood transfusions. As a Jehovah Witness she was not able to accept the treatment. The other doctors told her she would be dead in six months if she did not take the chemotherapy. She still refused and returned to our clinic for a holistic program.

As with all chronic patients, the first step was the candida cleanse. Again, this is done to aid in healing the immune system. Cancer is a systemic failure of the immune system and it is a well established fact that it is important for the patient's own immune system to begin to fight back. Normally, most people are exposed to cancer as tiny little errant cells. In a healthy immune system we respond to the threat and destroy the cancer cells on our own. In the case of cancer patients, their immune system was compromised and did not destroy the threat.

This can have a wide variety of root causes but in the end we ALWAYS and with no exceptions, find each cancer patient presenting extensive candida overgrowth. It is our job then, at the beginning, to aid the patient in reestablishing the intestinal environment. Once this is done than the patient has a higher likelihood of having a stronger immune system.

Once the 18 day candida cleanse is completed we then proceed with actually fighting the cancer. The patient remains on a vegan diet but at this point they begin to increase dramatically the percentage of raw, live food. We supply them with a wide variety of meal plans, recipes and nutrition charts so this does not become a boring diet.

We also being the holistic medication portion of the regimen. Colon and liver cleanses are done throughout the program along with herbal formulas utilizing Poke root, Red Raspberry tea, Milk thistle, blood cleanser formulas using Red Clover, and Thunder god vine root.

Thunder god vine root has been studied extensively out of China, Germany and even here in the states under Johns Hopkins University. Clinical trial studies seem to indicate that this herb out of China is able to begin the process of apoptosis with in 40 days. Apoptosis is the process by which cancer cells switch off their DNA and "commit suicide", so to speak.

With programs such as this kind, we ask the patient to return to the clinic once a month so we can check their progress, run vitals, run tests in house, all in an effort to monitor their treatments. We also regularly ran blood work on her cancer markers.

With each visit she reported feeling better and the masses, examined through ultrasound continued to shrink. Her cancer marker also continued to drop closer to the normal ranges. MRIs and CT scans were run about every six months.

At her last MRI scan along with ultrasound and blood work the local hospital declared no sign of the cancer any longer and to their surprise, her colon had "rebuilt itself".

Throughout her program she remained not only vegan but a high raw one and the results show in the spectacular healing the body can achieve through giving it want it naturally needs to heal. She recently came to me and stated she will never go back to her old diet again.

Something we try and teach each patient is that the body is an amazing creation and that it is designed with a built in "blueprint" if given the opportunity, it will heal and repair itself. As a very famous Naturopathic doctor and Master herbalist, Dr. John Christopher, stated:

"There is no such thing as an incurable disease, only incurable people".

5.3 Where to go from here

As always, please share this information with your healthcare provider before proceeding on any form of self treatment.

NO SPECIAL DIET PLANS NEEDED

You may have noticed by now that there is little mentioned in the way of special recipes or menu plans for a specific disease. This is because, in my personal experience and that of 20 years as a doctor treating patients with a wide variety of chronic conditions, that it is not so much a special food here or there but a diet rich in living enzymes and micro-nutrients. A diet packed with vitamins and minerals and their accompanying enzymes, in their fresh, living state, have more value in healing the body than any medicine that exists today for the treatment of chronic disorders.

Now, having said that, I must state that I have seen in case after case, when treating cancer, that a raw, vegan diet with a very high percentage of the food intake being in the form of pure, fresh, raw juices is superior to anything else I have seen. My cancer patients are instructed to regularly drinks copious amounts of these juices, generally in the form of green drinks with carrot and beet added. My common joke is for the drink to be basically, a salad in a glass, lots of veggies from a wide variety of different colors, with some fruit added as well. My preference is that this be the lion's share of their diet, especially in cases where the cancer is late stage. I have seen miracles occur following this routine.

WATCH FOR THE DETOX

Another important point to make here is about experiencing a detox once you go onto a diet consisting largely of raw, living foods. I have heard from so many patients complaining how they felt worse on a living diet than they did before. For many, this was enough for them to quit and return back to their old ways. In almost every case, what they are experiencing is a lifetime of heavy metals, candida die-off, old metabolic sediment and old pharmaceuticals being purged from the tissues. As they reenter the blood stream you may feel such symptoms s fatigue, headaches, nausea, flu-like symptoms, anxiety and depression, mood swings and others.

We try and let the patients know this is just a temporary situation and if they will drink yet more juices they detox will pass more easily. I have seen cases verified through blood work, where an individual dumped back into the blood stream medications they had taken 40 years prior to the cleanse. Needless to say (but I will anyway), this can encourage one to proceed a bit more cautiously with the detox, especially in those with very serious, life-threatening illness, such as late stage cancer and such. It requires a greater amount of monitoring but I have seen it work in many patients over the years.

As in most cases, old drugs, pharmaceuticals, toxins, poisons, environmentals, heavy metals and such store in the fatty parts of the body. So, during a transition to a raw, vegan diet one invariably will lose weight. As the pounds are melted away, that can mean that these old toxins are then re-released back into the blood stream, bringing about a detox. Again, this is often the case of patients stating they feel worse with the diet change. As always, I let them know to maintain a large intake of fluids to cleanse the blood and to not give up. The worst is usually over in a few days.

But, those are are seriously overweight, they will very likely experience this detox over and over again as the weight drops off, as old toxins find their way back into the blood. But, as time goes by, the patient begins to notice that the severity of the detox lessens with each event and their overall health continually improves.

OK, WHERE TO NOW?

The sky is the limit. For myself, when I made the transition to a raw, vegan, living food based diet the changes I experienced in my health were both amazing and a little surprising at how fast they occurred. Being a doctor in a clinical environment it is easy to providers get sick on a weekly basis due to exposure to so much brought into the clinic. I too would get sick several times a year before I transitioned but since I switched to this diet illness is now a rarely and is usually duet to stress, self-inflicted. I would never caret o go back to a diet of dead, life-less food where most of the nutrients had to be replaced after the processing was done. My energy level is fantastic and I do very well on one meal a day.

Where you go from here is up to you. We all must take personal charge of our health and own it, no other doctor on Earth can do that for you. In the end, the only healer in your life is you.

Below is a list of wonderful resources you may want to consider to continue your education. I made great use of all of them in my practice and personal experiences.

VIDEOS:

- **Fat, Sick And Nearly Dead** website: https://www.rebootwithjoe.com/

Storyline
     100 pounds overweight, loaded up on steroids and suffering from a debilitating autoimmune disease, Joe Cross is at the end of his rope and the end of his hope. In the mirror he saw a 310lb man whose gut was bigger than a beach ball and a path laid out before him that wouldn't end well- with one foot already in the grave, the other wasn't far behind. FAT, SICK & NEARLY DEAD is an inspiring film that chronicles Joe's personal mission to regain his health. With doctors and conventional medicines unable to help long-term, Joe turns to the only option left, the body's ability to heal itself. He trades in the junk food and hits the road with juicer and generator in tow, vowing only to drink fresh fruit and vegetable juice for the next 60 days. Across 3,000 miles Joe has one goal in mind: To get off his pills and achieve a balanced lifestyle. While talking to more than 500 Americans about food, health and longevity, it's at a truck stop in Arizona where Joe meets a truck driver who suffers ...

- **Simply Raw: Reversing Diabetes in 30 Days** – Can be found on Amazon at https://www.amazon.com/Simply-Raw-Reversing-Diabetes-Days/dp/B001BKLCCS/ref=sr_1_2?keywords=Simply+raw&qid=1583089815&sr=8-2

Simply Raw: Reversing Diabetes in 30 Days is an independent documentary film that chronicles six Americans with diabetes who switch to a diet consisting entirely of vegan, organic, uncooked food in order to reverse disease without pharmaceutical medication.

The six are challenged to give up meat, dairy, sugar, alcohol, nicotine, caffeine, soda, junk food, fast food, processed food, packaged food, and even cooked food for 30 days. The film follows each participant's remarkable journey and captures the medical, physical, and emotional transformations brought on by this radical diet and lifestyle change. We witness moments of struggle, support, and hope as what is revealed, with startling clarity, is that diet can reverse disease and change lives.

The film highlights each of the six before they begin the program and we first meet them in their home environment with their families. Each participant speaks candidly about their struggle to manage their diabetes and how it has affected every aspect of their life, from work to home to their relationships.

- **Living on Live Food DVD.** Found on Amazon.

An up-close and personal session with Alissa Cohen! Watch and listen as Alissa prepares over 20 delicious, mouthwatering recipes. You will be sitting in on a 3 hour food preparation class and in-depth discussion of the raw and living food diet along with two of Alissa's clients. Witnessing this live, one on one, 3 hour presentation of the raw and living food diet (recipe prep, client interaction, questions and answers, etc...) is invaluable, not only for learning how to prepare raw and living food but also in catching the excitement and enthusiasm of how miraculous, life changing and fun this way of eating can be! Don't miss the finale which captures the amazing weight loss transformations of Nancy and Sharon after their 30 day challenge to stay 100% raw! Alissa, All I can say is...WOW!!! The 2 recipes you sent me were great! Great tasting and very easy to make. My girlfriend couldn't believe the torte was raw! Thanks. I can't wait until the Living on Live Food book/DVD come out. If all your recipes are this easy to make, going raw should be illegal! - Chris Bellinger The recipes on these DVDs are in printed form in the Living on Live Food book. There are 2 DVD's in this set.

BOOKS:

- **Living on Live Food Book. By Alissa Cohen**

Living on Live Food teaches you what a raw and living food diet is and how to get started immediately! But that's not all, this motivational book also covers such topics as: addiction to cooked foods, changing your thought process, being social while staying healthy, enzymes, acid-alkaline balance, strategies and techniques, matters beyond food... plus so much more. 290 Recipes and detailed 4-week plan complete with menu, shopping lists and meal preparation instructions. 15 compelling real-life success stories with amazing before and after photographs. "You will see results! Not within years, or months, or even weeks, but within days! Does this sound like I'm promising a lot? I am! But I'm not exaggerating. You'll believe me almost from the instant you start eating this way. It's a miracle just waiting to happen to you." (600 pages. Paper)

- **Ani's RAW FOOD ESSENTIALS by Ani Phyo**

Want to go raw, but not sure how to start? *Ani's Raw Food Essentials* offers easy transitional recipes--using the equipment you already have in your kitchen. Looking for innovative meals that are healthy and delicious? Ani offers everything from comfort classics like nachos and burgers to more gourmet dishes like risotto, angel hair pasta, and her you-won't-believe-they're-raw desserts. *Ani's Raw Food Essentials* once again proves that you don't have to sacrifice taste to reap the benefits of raw foods and a greener lifestyle.

- **The 80/10/10 Diet by Dr. Douglas N. Graham**

After more than 5 years of intensive work the definitive guide to the 80/10/10 Diet is here! Get your hands on the latest book by Dr. Douglas Graham, The 80/10/10 Diet: Balancing Your Health, Your Weight, and Your Life One Luscious Bite at a Time. If you have struggled with staying raw, would like to lose weight, or change your life for the better, look no further than this groundbreaking book.

FURTHER YOU HEALTH EDUCATION:

This book is six in the **Healing Naturally** book series by Dr. Earendil Spindelilus. Below is a short description of the rest of the series and how they can benefit your life by teaching you how to care for your own health and that of your families:

- *A Holistic Approach To Healing Lyme Disease* - The purpose of this book is to offer an alternative treatment for both acute and chronic Lyme disease. To date there are currently 300,000 new cases of Lyme reported in the United States each year. There are six times the reported new cases of HIV. It is the new pandemic of this century. Sadly, most doctors today are either not Lyme-literate or prefer to choose the conventional approach to treatment which is simply symptomatic with high doses of antibiotics. This method has been proven to offer no cure for this disorder and in the end bankrupts most patients. This book will explain in detail the etiology of Lyme, current accepted conventional protocols, along with a treatment plan I have been using in practice for over 20 years. I will also be discussing successful case histories where patients were cured and remain so to this day.
- *Case Histories From A Successful Naturopathic Medical Clinic* - The purpose of this book is to offer hope for an alternative treatment for chronic disease. The information contained describes in a small detail some of the work and case histories I have personally witnessed in my 20+ years of practice as an alternative healthcare provider. You will find a wide variety of cases ranging from simple cuts and wounds to serious auto-immune disorders such as Multiple Sclerosis and type 1 diabetes along with successful treatments for cancer.
- *A Complete Body Repair* - Throughout my 20+ years of practice one of the most frustrating complaints I hear from new patients is the lack of a proper diagnosis. For most, they have spent years going from one doctor to another, sometimes trying both conventional and alternative methods, to no avail. They come to the clinic sad, angry, frustrated and bitter at the medical community and have little hope remaining. This is the common attitude I am faced with each day. Within this book I will cover each of these topics in detail, describing what they

are, the causes, how to diagnose, conditions caused by them, conventional treatments and how to successfully treat holistically.
- ***Holistic First-Aid*** - I can say that while technology seems to have made lives easier, I would not say it has made them better. A case in point is the lack of knowledge these days in the proper care and feeding of emergency situations. There was a time when most folks had at least a rudimentary understanding of first aid care and could handle most situations on their own. Most families or villages had a skilled healer in the community who knew enough to intervene when an accident occurred. In this book we will learn about the natural treatment for such issues as burns, bleeding both minor and more severe, various types of poisonings, broken bone after care, snake bites, immediate life saving care for a heart attack or stroke victim, eye injuries, minor dental complaints and many more. You also learn how to make your own medications.
- ***The Handbook Of Holistic Healing*** - With the great success of the Healing Naturally book series, we decided to combine all four current books into one complete handbook at a discounted price. All of the information from the full set is included along with a bonus chapter for helping you treat your companion animals at home! Within the pages of this book you can learn to care for the most common root causes of most disease.

About The Author

Dr. Earendil M. Spindelilus D.N.M., M.H., C.R. - Traditional Naturopath, Holistic Practitioner, Clinical Master Herbalist, Certified Nutritionist, Certified Reflexology, Member of Plant Savers of America, Member of American Botanical Council.

I hold a Doctorate degree in Natural Medicine. I have also been a lecturer since 1999. Board Certified Diplomate of Natural Medicine. Member of the American Council of Holistic Medicine. I am also a raw, vegan doctor and nutritionist and have been using these recipes and protocols mentioned in this book with my patients for over 20 years.

I have always had a deep and abiding interest in the Plant Kingdom. Even very young I loved the way the herbs held the mystery of healing within them and how I could learn about them. I traveled around the world learning from different cultures their own unique floras and how they incorporated them into their daily lives. With each new herb I learned how special the world is and how Nature supplies us with all we need. In the 1990s I decided to take my education further and enrolled in the School and Natural Healing, the College of Herbal Medicine. I graduated in 1999 with my Master Herbalist. I have also studied with the New Eden School of Natural Medicine where I completed my Doctorate in Natural Medicine. To date, my wife and I have run two medical centers for natural healing. It has always been a great joy meeting with our patients. We are all meant to live a happy, healthy life and when we allow our body to perform it's innate ability to heal itself then this can happen. I am also a past board member of the Reflexology Association of California as well as a published author/writer of numerous holistic books and articles. I am also a past host of a holistic radio show.

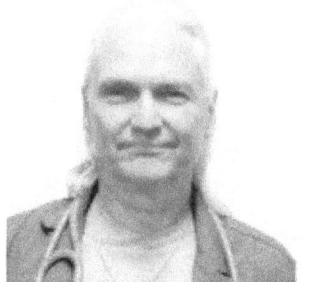

www.ingramcontent.com/pod-product-compliance
Lightning Source LLC
Chambersburg PA
CBHW071349210526
45465CB00001B/35